Migraine and other headaches

YOUR QUESTIONS ANSWERED

Commissioning Editor: Ellen Green
Project development and management: Fiona Conn
Design direction: Jayne Jones, George Ajayi, Keith Kail

Migraine and other headaches

YOUR QUESTIONS ANSWERED

Andrew J Dowson
MBBS MRCGP
Director of the King's Headache Service,
King's College Hospital,
London, UK

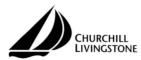

CHURCHILL
LIVINGSTONE

EDINBURGH LONDON NEW YORK PHILADELPHIA ST LOUIS SYDNEY TORONTO 2003

CHURCHILL LIVINGSTONE
An imprint of Elsevier Science Limited

First published 2003

ISBN 0 443 07339 2

British Library Cataloguing in Publication Data
A catalogue record for this book is available from the British Library

Library of Congress Cataloging in Publication Data
A catalog record for this book is available from the Library of Congress

Note
Medical knowledge is constantly changing. As new information becomes
available, changes in treatment, procedures, equipment and the use of
drugs become necessary. The author and the publishers have taken care
to ensure that the information given in this text is accurate and up to date.
However, readers are strongly advised to confirm that the information,
especially with regard to drug usage, complies with the latest legislation
and standards of practice.

your source for books,
journals and multimedia
in the health sciences
www.elsevierhealth.com

Printed in China by RDC Group Limited

Contents

About this book

Headache can at times be daunting to manage in the primary care setting. There is a widespread belief that it is a trivial condition. Patients rarely consult their doctor just for headache, either not consulting at all or mentioning it in passing at the end of a consultation for another condition. The doctor is often given little medical education on headache and is presented with what can seem to be a bewildering variety of conditions to diagnose and manage. Justifiably, they are most concerned with the exclusion or treatment of sinister, secondary headaches that may be life-threatening to the patient. However, most headaches encountered in primary care are benign and straightforward to diagnose and manage. With a little education, many of the necessary management skills can be conducted by a practice nurse or pharmacist.

Headache is a very common condition. Almost all of the population (96%) suffers from headache at some time in their lives and approximately 70% have headache on at least a monthly basis. The vast majority of these disorders are due to benign primary headaches that resolve spontaneously without treatment but which nevertheless can significantly limit the lifestyle of the sufferer. These headaches can be intermittent or chronic in nature. The proportion of people who have sinister, secondary headaches is incredibly small. Headaches most frequently encountered in primary care include migraine, tension-type headache, short, sharp headache, cluster headache, chronic daily headache and sinus headaches and other causes of facial pain.

This short book uses a 'question and answer' format to provide the information necessary for the primary care doctor to manage migraine (and other common headaches) effectively in their practices. The book is also designed for use by practice nurses and pharmacists, who form an integral part of the primary healthcare team for headache.

Chapter 1 contains an overview of the main types of headaches encountered in primary care, some of their causes and their distribution in the various age groups in the population.

Chapter 2 covers the current state of knowledge of migraine; its epidemiology, natural history, illness burden, aetiology, pathogenesis and relationship to other headaches.

Chapter 3 covers the practical diagnosis of migraine and its differentiation from other headache disorders.

Chapter 4 provides an evidence-based review of the clinical profiles of available medications used for the treatment of migraine.

Chapter 5 investigates current practices of managing migraine and their pitfalls, together with a practical guide for the overall management of migraine in the primary care setting.

Chapter 6 provides the same information as chapter 5 for the nonmigraine headaches.

Chapter 7 looks into the practical details of how headache management can be organised in primary care by the setting up of a 'primary care headache team'.

Finally, Chapter 8 takes a look into the future, examining new strategies and treatment modalities for migraine that are on the horizon.

All chapters (except Chapter 8) include questions that are frequently asked by patients and provide answers written at a level that the layperson can understand.

The writing of this book has involved a review and synthesis of material contained in hundreds of published books, articles and congress presentations. However, for ease of use only a short reference list follows the text. This contains key publications and textbooks that the interested physician can use as a starting point for further investigation. Also included are publications designed for primary care physicians and patients that are accessible but comprehensive.

Two appendices are provided at the back of the book. Appendix 1 is a list of the available drugs for migraine, with details of their formulations, dosing schedules, side effects and other relevant material. Appendix 2 contains details of professional organisations and websites designed for the headache specialist, primary care physician and patient. These sites contain a wealth of further information that can be easily accessed.

The book is not specifically designed to be read from beginning to end but to be dipped into for the specific information required. To help with this, great emphasis is placed on cross-referencing of linked items, so that all the information relevant to a topic can be quickly accessed. However, I hope that the book is organised in such a way that it can be read from cover to cover for those who wish to do so.

AJD

ACKNOWLEDGEMENT
The author wishes to thank Dr Pete Blakeborough of Alpha-Plus Medical Communications Ltd for his help in the preparation of this book.

How to use this book

'Migraine: Your Questions Answered' is a concise guide that aims to provide expert information at your fingertips concerning the management of migraine and other headaches in primary care. It is targeted for the information needs of primary care physicians and other primary care professionals who care for sufferers of these disorders, providing practical, evidence-based guidelines for their care.

The format of the book is highly structured. Usually, each topic has an introductory question that sets up the discussion point, followed by a series of questions and answers that examine it in detail. Tables, figures, boxes and icons are used to draw the reader to important points.

ICONS

Using the icons will help to access important information quickly. The following icons are used to identify particular types of information:

 highlights information important to clinical practice

 highlights side effect information.

PATIENT QUESTIONS

At the end of relevant chapters there are sections of frequently asked patient questions, with easy-to-understand answers aimed at the non-medical reader. These questions are also listed at the end of the book.

Headache in primary care

HEADACHES

1.1 Who gets headaches?

Virtually everyone experiences headache at some time in their lives. However, the proportion of the population who experience regular headaches is surprisingly large, with about 70% of people reporting one or more headaches per month. Headache is not a static disorder; the types of headache change through peoples' lives. Children, adolescents, and young, middle-aged and elderly people all have their own distinctive types of headache. Headache may be associated with specific physiological processes (e.g. the menstrual period in women) and is often reported by patients associated with common illnesses (e.g. infectious diseases).

It may be thought from this that headache would be encountered commonly by the primary care physician. However, this is not the case and relatively few consultations are for headache only. Patients will often attend the clinic for other disorders and only mention (if at all) that they have headaches after the consultation when they are leaving the surgery. Such patients form a significant proportion of the 'heartsink' patients in the physician's practice. Primary care physicians also tend to have little formal education about headache and little time to deal with each patient. The end result is that the patient with headache is frequently marginalised, both by healthcare professionals and through their own actions.

1.2 Who do headache sufferers first contact for advice and care?

It has to be said that the majority of headache sufferers probably do not consult any healthcare professional for advice and care, relying, if at all, on friends and family for advice. They either cope as best they can without treatment or self-medicate with the plethora of over-the-counter (OTC) painkilling medications available at pharmacists, supermarkets and even convenience stores. Some will also use homeopathic and herbal remedies available at health food shops. Of these, paracetamol and aspirin and other nonsteroidal anti-inflammatory drugs (NSAIDs) are most frequently bought and used. If these do not work, patients may graduate towards stronger combination therapies available at pharmacists where codeine is added to the aspirin or paracetamol.

It may only be when the patient has exhausted these proprietary medications that they will go to a healthcare professional for advice. Even then, the primary care physician is unlikely to be their first port of call. Headache sufferers are more likely to consult their pharmacist, practice nurse or an alternative practitioner than their primary care physician. The end result is that the headache sufferer that the physician sees for the first time is likely to have had their symptoms for a long time and may have exhausted all available alternative options.

1.3 What are the pathways of medical care for headache?

The formal approach to seeking medical care is for the patient to initially consult their primary care physician, who instigates a diagnostic evaluation before prescribing appropriate therapy. If the primary care physician is uncertain of the diagnosis, diagnoses a serious condition, or finds that repeated therapy has little effect on the condition, they are likely to refer the patient to a specialist physician for further evaluation. This pattern of care does take place in patients with headache. Some patients do consult their primary care physician, who may refer them to either a neurologist or headache specialist if necessary.

However, this classic approach to care is often not used for headache. Many healthcare professionals other than physicians may be contacted by headache sufferers for care, including:

- Pharmacists: for general advice and over-the-counter medications
- Opticians: for headache related to eye strain
- Dentists: for headache associated with the jaws and face
- Practice nurses: at the various clinics that they run
- School nurses: for headaches in children
- Chiropractors and other 'alternative' healthcare providers.

The end result is that the primary care physician often has to deal with severely affected patients who may be difficult to treat.

1.4 What types of headache are encountered in primary care?

Types of headache encountered in primary care

Migraine (*see Qs 1.5–12*)

Tension-type headache (TTH) is a very common acute, intermittent headache, but is generally not disabling and is relatively easily managed. About 50% of the population may be affected by these headaches on a monthly basis.

Short, sharp headaches are acute, intermittent headaches that are much less common than migraine and tension-type headache, and often triggered by cold. For this reason, they are often called 'ice cream' or 'ice pick' headaches.

Cluster headache is a rare condition that can be acute or chronic in nature, and mostly affects men. It is characterised by relatively short-lived (15 minutes to 3 hours), but intensely painful headaches that occur several times a day for periods of weeks, months or on a constant, daily basis. This condition is only present in about 0.25% of people.

Chronic daily headaches (CDH), as the name suggests, comprise daily or near-daily headaches that last for more than 4 hours and are often linked to analgesic overuse or head injury. They are relatively common, affecting about 5% of the population, and usually arise from a primary, acute headache disorder.

Facial pain: Sinusitis headaches are caused by infection of the cranial sinuses. They are relatively uncommon. However, they are often confused with migraine and tension-type headaches. Other types of facial pain include trigeminal neuralgia (short, paroxysmal facial pain usually seen in the elderly), post-herpetic neuralgia (paroxysmal pain after an eruption of herpes Zoster) and temperomandibular joint dysfunction.

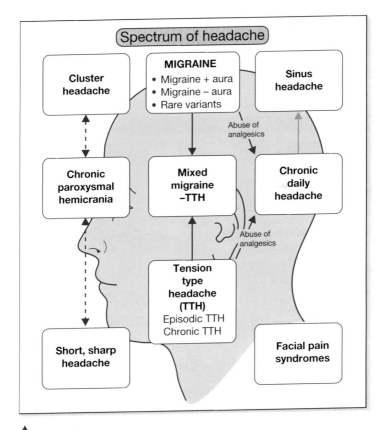

Fig. 1.1 Headache subtypes that may be encountered in primary care.

Most headaches that physicians deal with in primary care are the benign subtypes of migraine and chronic daily headache. Even though it is the commonest headache, tension-type headache is encountered infrequently in normal clinical practice, as patients rarely consult for this condition. Trigeminal neuralgia, postherpetic neuralgia and temporomandibular joint dysfunction, although not common, will also be encountered on a more or less regular basis (*Fig. 1.1*).

Patients also frequently consult for headaches that they describe as 'sinus headaches'. As we shall see, these headaches are relatively uncommon and are frequently diagnosed for what are in fact migraine or tension-type headaches.

Patients are also frequently concerned that their headache may be due to a brain tumour or other sinister cause. Such headaches are in fact extremely rare and the patients will usually have migraine or chronic daily headache.

The primary care physician will only rarely see the headache subtypes of cluster headache and short, sharp headache and may never see patients with some of the rare migraine manifestations.

MIGRAINE

1.5   What is migraine?

> **Symptoms of migraine**
>
> Migraine is a clinical syndrome consisting of attacks of multiple symptoms, which occur in an episodic fashion over decades of a sufferer's life, attacks being separated by symptom-free intervals. These include
>
> - headache
> - nausea
> - sensory sensitivity
> - muscle pain
> - cognitive disruptions
> - autonomic symptoms

Migraine attacks are disruptive to the sufferer's lifestyle, and sufferers experience poorer quality of life during their attacks than the general healthy population. Genetic factors may determine the threshold for migraine sensitivity.

Migraine is the most frequently seen disabling headache in primary care. Until recently, relatively little was known about its causes, prevalence, distribution in society and impact on sufferers and the nation's economy. There have perhaps been more incorrect 'myths' concerning migraine than any other medical condition. However, in the past decade or so, there has been an explosion of new information concerning the condition. We now know what causes migraine, its natural history, the people who are affected and the extent of their suffering. This has coincided with the development and marketing of new, effective migraine therapies that have the potential to transform migraine treatment.

1.6   What are the main subtypes of migraine?

There are two main subtypes of migraine:

- Migraine with aura (previously known as *classical* migraine)
- Migraine without aura (previously known as *common* migraine).

These two subtypes are associated with similar headache and other symptoms, except that migraine with aura also has a phase of reversible sensory symptoms in the time (usually 1 hour) preceding the development of headache. These are known as auras, and include visual changes such as zigzag lines, blurred vision, flashing lights or scotoma (holes in the vision). However, a variety of other symptoms may also occur such as word-salading (words being mixed up), dizziness, tingling, numbness, sensory loss and limb weakness. Approximately 10% of migraine sufferers experience attacks of migraine with aura, although they usually also have attacks of migraine without aura. The presence of aura is not predictive of attack severity. Attacks of migraine without aura may be equally or even more severe than attacks of migraine with aura.

There are certain rare subtypes of migraine that are characterised by atypical aura symptoms. These conditions are considered later in this section (*see* Q 1.12).

1.7   What is 'migrainous' headache?

Migrainous headache is a technical term used in the classification of migraine subtypes. It refers to a headache that in all respects but one meets the diagnostic criteria for migraine (*see* Q 3.4). For the purposes of primary care practice, migrainous headache should be considered as normal migraine and managed accordingly.

1.8   What is menstrual migraine?

Migraine is 2–3 times more prevalent in women than in men after puberty and is often associated with the menstrual period in women. Menstrual migraine has been defined in several ways but the consensus today is for attacks that begin during the time period from the day prior to the start of menstruation and day 3 of menstruation to be classified as menstrual migraine. Such attacks are common and more than 50% of women with migraine report an association between migraine and menstruation, although in most cases they also have migraine attacks outside the menstrual period. Studies indicate that menstrual migraine attacks are the result of oestrogen withdrawal in the late luteal phase of the normal menstrual cycle but other factors such as prostaglandin release have also been implicated.

It is widely considered that menstrual migraine attacks are more severe and less responsive to treatment than nonmenstrual attacks but recent studies have tended to refute this. Despite this, menstrual migraine attacks tend to be treated in the same way as nonmenstrual attacks in clinical practice. They are treated with standard acute therapies and, if necessary, with specific short-term prophylactic treatments such as oestrogen supplements given during the perimenstrual period.

1.9 What is early-morning migraine?

Migraine is unpredictable in its occurrence and attacks can start at any time of the day. However, many patients report attacks that are fully developed on waking up in the morning and they tend to be woken up by the headache. These attacks are particularly severe and difficult to treat, as the patient has no chance to take preventative steps before the attack starts or when it is in its early, milder stages.

It is important that patients prone to these migraine attacks have a ready supply of effective abortive treatments to hand so that they can treat the attack as soon as possible. It is unrealistic to expect such patients to be able to attend the physician's surgery for treatment.

1.10 What are the features of migraine in children?

Headache is a common complaint in children and adolescents, and may be due to migraine, tension-type headache or other causes. Studies show that between half to three-quarters of children aged 12–17 years experience one or more headaches per month, a frequency similar to that reported for adults. About 15% of children are likely to experience a migraine attack or chronic tension-type headaches before the age of 15. It is important that the physician considers headache as a cause of childhood morbidity, as it may lead to absence from school.

In general, migraine manifests in a similar way in children as it does in adults. Most sufferers (about 70%) have a positive family history of migraine. However, aura symptoms may be less common in children than in adults. Prodrome (premonitory) symptoms and trigger factors are commonly present (*see Qs 2.14 and 2.46*). The characteristic features of childhood migraine are:

- Attacks that last 1–4 hours, compared with 4–72 hours in adults
- Frontal headache, compared with predominantly one-sided headache in adults

■ Associated nausea and vomiting and abdominal pain
■ Associated photophobia and phonophobia.

During the attack, sufferers often retire to their rooms, complaining of photophobia and phonophobia, and wanting to go to sleep. They then usually fall asleep for 2–6 hours and wake up with the attack resolved.

Migraine can start at a very early age, with an average age of onset of about 5 years. It is equally common in boys and girls up to puberty but becomes markedly more common in girls after this point.

1.11 Can migraine manifest in children in different ways to how it does in adults?

Migraine in younger children can manifest itself with symptoms quite different from those reported by older children and adults:

■ Episodes of paroxysmal vertigo may start to occur in children between 2–6 years of age but are reported in all age groups. These attacks are brief and sudden, lasting a few minutes only, but do recur. The child may lose balance and be unable to walk during the attacks.
■ Young children may also experience episodes of cyclical vomiting, lasting about 1 day and occurring every 1–2 months. These attacks are often precipitated by travel. The clinical features of cyclical vomiting overlap to a large extent with those of migraine.
■ In older preadolescent children, gastrointestinal symptoms may be indicative of migraine. Children may have episodes of paroxysmal abdominal pain, without the headache – such attacks are known as 'abdominal migraine'.
■ Episodes of short-lasting, recurrent limb pain are common in children and, where they are not due to injury, may be indicative of childhood migraine.
■ In general, children with migraine may be more prone to travel sickness, sleep disturbances, be more fearful and prone to frustration and be less physically strong than the general population. They may present as being emotionally rigid, with repressed anger and aggression.

These symptoms are frequently misunderstood by parents and physicians and may be blamed on stress, or as the child malingering to avoid going to school. It is important to realise their true cause, so avoiding much physical and emotional suffering. As the child moves into adolescence, these symptoms tend to disappear, to be replaced by the symptoms typical of migraine.

1.12 What are the rare migraine manifestations?

There are several rare subtypes of migraine with aura or headache symptoms that differ from those normally encountered in clinical practice.

■ *Prolonged aura*: The aura may be prolonged in some patients, lasting from more than 60 minutes up to 7 days, although most sufferers have normal duration auras for most of their attacks.

■ *Familial hemiplegic migraine*: Patients have this condition if their aura symptoms include hemiparesis, which may be prolonged, and a first-degree relative who has the same condition.

■ *Basilar migraine*: In this subtype, aura symptoms are present that clearly originate from the brainstem or the occipital lobes, including visual symptoms in both the temporal and nasal fields of both eyes, dysarthria, vertigo, tinnitus, decreased hearing, double vision, ataxia, bilateral paraesthesias and pareses and a decreased level of consciousness.

■ *Attacks of migraine aura* without subsequent development of headache are relatively common, especially as migraine sufferers get older.

■ *Retinal migraine*: In this condition, repeated attacks of monocular scotoma or blindness lasting less than 1 hour are associated with headache.

■ *Migrainous infarction*: In this condition, aura symptoms are prolonged past a 7-day period and/or are associated with a cerebral infarction. Shorter-lasting auras may also be indicative of neurological deficit. Aura-type symptoms lasting up to 24 hours may be associated with transient ischaemic attacks (TIAs), while those lasting between 24 hours and 7 days may be associated with reversible ischaemic neurological deficit (RIND).

■ *Ophthalmoplegic migraine*: In this very rare condition in children aged 6–12 years, attacks of headache are very prolonged and associated with paresis of one or more cranial ocular nerves resulting in weakness in one of the eye muscles.

■ *Status migrainosus*: In this condition, the headache phase of the migraine attacks lasts > 72 hours, despite treatment. Headache-free intervals of up to 4 hours may occur during this time. It is usually associated with prolonged drug use.

These conditions may in fact not be migraine manifestations but symptomatic of underlying serious pathology. The differential diagnosis of these conditions is discussed later in this book (*see Q 3.8*). However, these conditions will be encountered rarely, if at all, by the primary care physician.

NONMIGRAINE HEADACHES

1.13 What are the secondary (sinister) headaches?

The vast majority of the headaches seen in primary care are benign primary headaches. Several illnesses also produce headaches as part of their symptom complexes but in most cases these are relatively minor conditions. Some of these are dealt with later.

Serious illnesses that produce sinister headaches

Sinister headaches arise as a side effect of serious and life-threatening illnesses and are rarely seen in primary care. They include:

- Meningitis and other infections
- Subarachnoid haemorrhages following head injury, pre-existing aneurisms or vascular malformations
- Cranial arteritis, due to inflammation of the cranial arteries
- Primary brain tumours
- Cerebral metastases
- Cerebral abscesses caused by bacterial, fungal or parasitic infections
- Strokes and transient ischaemic attacks.

The diagnosis of sinister headaches is discussed later in this book (*see Q 3.27*). The role of the primary care physician in these cases is usually to identify patients with high risk of having sinister headaches and referring them for specialist care.

1.14 What is tension-type headache?

Tension-type headache (sometimes called muscle-contraction headache) is the commonest headache experienced by the general population, with about half of all people having such headaches on at least a monthly basis. Interestingly, sufferers rarely consult their physicians for tension-type headache, preferring to manage the condition without outside help. This may be because, unlike migraine, tension-type headaches are of low impact, even though they tend to be of longer duration.

Tension-type headaches may arise due to the body's response to emotional or physical stimuli, such as:

- Stress
- Anxiety
- Depression
- Emotional conflicts
- Anger
- Fatigue.

Such triggers lead to a physiological response of reflex dilatation of the external cranial arteries and contraction of skeletal muscles in the head, face and neck, leading to the headache.

Tension-type headaches are usually bilateral, steady, nonpulsating and located in the forehead, temples and back of the head or neck. Patients commonly describe the headache as being an ache that is tight, vice-like, pressing or sore. Tension-type headache is more common in women than in men and can occur at any age, but usually starts between the ages of 20 and 40 years. The headache may be episodic (occurring on < 15 days per month) or chronic (occurring on ≥ 15 days per month).

1.15   What are short, sharp headaches?

Short, sharp headaches are very short-lived, very severe and often described as 'like a flash of lightning'. Most of these headaches last only up to 30 seconds but can recur several times a day. The headache is usually centred on one eye and patients may feel bruised after the pain has resolved. These headaches can be triggered by eating ice cream or other cold foods, and are commonly called 'ice cream' or 'ice pick' headaches.

Patients with short, sharp headaches are often young to middle-aged adults. They are not commonly seen in primary care but will be encountered occasionally. For example, approximately 5% of patients referred to a UK secondary care headache clinic had this type of headache.

Sometimes these headaches last longer than 30 seconds. They are referred to as 'chronic paroxysmal hemicrania' if the headache continues for longer than 3 minutes and diffusely affects one side of the head.

1.16   What is cluster headache?

Cluster headache is a rare but very painful condition, characterised by intermittent attacks of excruciatingly severe unilateral headache, accompanied by symptoms such as conjunctival infection, lacrimation, nasal congestion, rhinorrhoea, forehead and facial sweating, miosis, ptosis and eyelid oedema. The headache is sudden in onset, frequently occurs around the eyes, and is often described as throbbing or pulsating, and constant or boring in nature. Cluster headaches last for an average of 45 minutes (ranging from 15 to 180 minutes) and are frequent, ranging from one every other day to eight times daily. Unlike with migraine, patients tend to be restless, upright and move about during their attacks.

Unlike migraine, cluster headache is more common in men than in women, with 3.5–7 times more men than women affected. The condition is encountered rarely in primary care, as only about 0.4% of men and 0.08% of women have the condition. Cluster headache usually starts between the ages of 20 and 40 years and patients usually do not have a family history of the condition.

Cluster headache may be episodic or chronic. Episodic cluster headache occurs for weeks or months, interspersed by months to years of remission from symptoms. Patients with chronic cluster headache have their attacks for more than 1 year, with pain-free periods of < 14 days. Most patients (80–90%) have the episodic form of the condition.

1.17 What is chronic daily headache?

Chronic daily headache is a descriptive rather than a diagnostic term for headaches that occur for more than 4 hours on more than 15 days per month. Many different classifications have been used for chronic daily headache, which can lead to confusion. Among the most commonly used terms are:

- Daily or near-daily headaches
- Chronic migraine
- Transformed migraine
- Chronic tension-type headache
- New persistent daily headache
- Medication misuse headache
- Hemicrania continua
- Analgesic-dependent headache.

These headaches are called 'chronic daily headaches' in this book. However, their classification is under review by the International Headache Society (IHS) and a new nomenclature may be introduced soon. Perhaps the most useful definition for chronic daily headache is when headache is present on the majority of days for a period of 6 months or longer, characterised by a combination of background tension-type headaches with migraine superimposed over this. Chronic tension-type headache and chronic migraine are also seen on their own.

Chronic daily headache is relatively common, affecting about 4% of the general adult population and about 1–2% of children. It can occur at all ages, from as young as 5 years to as old as over 80 years. Unlike migraine, chronic daily headache is twice as prevalent in men as in women. Symptoms can continue for decades if treatment is not initiated. In general practice, about 50% of patients consulting for headache have chronic headache.

1.18 What are the different clinical presentations of chronic daily headache?

Chronic daily headache presents in a variety of forms (*Fig.1. 2*). The balance between the tension-type headaches and migraine varies from patient to patient:

- At one extreme, some patients experience tension-type headaches only (chronic tension-type headache).
- When migraine attacks occur, their frequency varies greatly. Some patients have tension-type headaches (stiffness in the neck and shoulders) all the time, with a migraine attack once every 2–3 months.

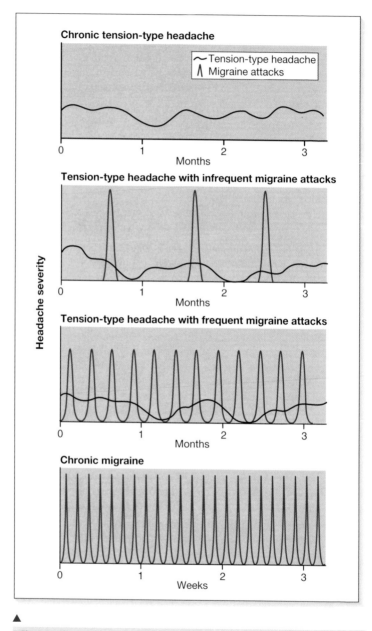

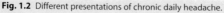

Fig. 1.2 Different presentations of chronic daily headache.

Patients may have more frequent migraine attacks, on a monthly, weekly, or even daily basis.

■ At the other extreme, patients may have daily, or near-daily, migraine attacks without significant tension-type headaches.

1.19 Can head and neck injury cause headaches?

Head and neck injuries frequently lead to headache, which may be acute, chronic or related to concussion. Up to half of patients with closed-head injuries experience headache post trauma. The headaches may present as tension-type headache, migraine, occipital neuralgia or with dysautonomic symptoms.

The commonest form of neck injury is whiplash following a car accident. An acute, dull headache may develop in the hours or days after the accident, which usually resolves within a few weeks. However, sometimes the pain persists and a chronic, severe, widespread pain develops (the full whiplash syndrome). The pain is worst in the mornings, during physical or mental exertion and on moving the neck. Previous head and neck injuries have been shown to be clear risk factors for the development of chronic daily headache.

1.20 Does misuse of alcohol and drugs cause headaches?

Headaches are often associated with the intake of recreational drugs, the clearest example being the hangover headache following alcohol intoxication. However, many prescribed drugs are associated with headache as an adverse event, particularly during the initial stages of treatment. Such symptoms tend to disappear with continued treatment. Headache may also be reported when the drug is overdosed.

A particularly insidious drug-related headache is caused by the overuse of headache medications. Patients who develop frequent headaches often find that they need to increase their dosage of painkilling medications due to the development of tolerance. This can lead to a rebound phenomenon, where the headache is relieved transiently with the painkiller but returns rapidly, necessitating a further dose of medication. The end result is the development of a particularly disabling form of chronic daily headache related to analgesic overdose. Indeed, there seem to be two groups of patients with chronic daily headache, those with analgesic dependence and those without.

Drugs that can cause analgesic dependence include simple and opiate analgesics, and the ergots. Codeine is particularly associated with analgesic dependence. There is some conjecture that overuse of triptans may lead to dependence but this is far from proven as yet. In almost all cases, the offending drug needs to be withdrawn before this type of headache can resolve.

1.21 What is cranial arteritis?

Cranial arteritis involves inflammation of the arteries of the head. The arteries become thickened, stop pulsating, are tender to the touch and the skin over the artery becomes red. In most patients, cranial arteritis is associated with a bilateral or unilateral continuous headache, with exacerbations caused by activities like hair brushing, which is particularly severe over the affected arteries. Pain in the muscles of the jaw may also occur when chewing — this is known as 'jaw claudication'. Cranial arteritis affects people over the age of 50 years and is more common in women than men.

1.22 What is sinus headache?

Infections of the sinuses may cause headaches, particularly acute sinusitis, where the infection lasts from 1 day to 3 weeks. Symptoms include headache and/or facial pain over the sinuses together with an acute febrile illness and a purulent discharge. In the absence of these latter two symptoms, the headache is much more likely to be due to migraine or tension-type headache.

The site of the pain varies according to the location of infection:

- Maxillary sinusitis pain is mostly in the cheek, gums, teeth and upper jaw
- Ethmoid sinusitis pain is between the eyes, with eye tenderness that is aggravated by eye movement
- Frontal sinusitis causes pain in the forehead
- Sphenoidal sinusitis pain is often at the vertex, or in or behind the eyes

Sinus headaches usually have a dull, aching quality that is worsened by sudden movements or by bending over.

1.23 What other types of facial pain are there?

Other common types of facial pain may be caused by trigeminal neuralgia, postherpetic neuralgia and temporomandibular joint dysfunction.

TRIGEMINAL NEURALGIA

Trigeminal neuralgia is an acute, short-lived, severe, paroxysmal pain of the facial or frontal regions along the divisions of the trigeminal nerve. The pain is unilateral, sudden, intensely severe, sharp, superficial, stabbing or burning in quality and may cause twitching of the facial muscles. However, it can also present as a sustained, deep, dull ache. The pain lasts from a few seconds to < 2 minutes, and between attacks the patients has no symptoms. Attacks are often triggered by washing, shaving, talking or brushing the teeth. Trigeminal neuralgia is the most common neurological syndrome in the elderly and is two to three times more common in women than in men.

POSTHERPETIC NEURALGIA

Postherpetic neuralgia occurs after an eruption of Herpes zoster. The pain often starts during the acute rash phase but is particularly problematic if it persists after the eruption has cleared. In this case, symptoms include a constant, deep, unilateral pain with repetitive stabs or needle-prick sensations. Any light touch can trigger the pain and also cause itching.

This type of neuralgia is most common in the elderly and can persist for months or years. It is associated with depression and dependency problems and is extremely disabling for patients. There can also be problems in diagnosing the original herpes infection, as the rash can be mild or invisible (e.g. a lesion in the eardrum).

TEMPOROMANDIBULAR JOINT DYSFUNCTION

Dysfunction of one of the temporomandibular joints can lead to pain in the upper part of the head on the affected side, limitation in jaw movement, muscle tenderness and joint crepitus. The cause is probably muscle spasms in the jaw. Episodes of jaw clenching may lead to tension-type headaches, while teeth grinding when asleep can lead to migraine attacks on wakening.

1.24 Does eye strain cause headache?

Weakness in the eye muscles, defects in eye focusing or sustained muscle contraction while trying to maintain normal vision may all cause headaches. The headaches tend to occur during close, sustained work, such as reading, working at a computer, sewing and similar activities. The headache often manifests at the end of a day of accommodating working muscles. Symptoms tend to be:

- Discomfort and heaviness around the eyes
- Pain starting over and around the eyes
- Pain gradually increasing in severity and radiating to the forehead and temples
- A blurring of vision.

Eye strain may occur and lead to headache at any time of life. It is common in children before they are prescribed spectacles and in middle-aged people as their eyesight changes with age.

1.25 Does high blood pressure cause headache?

Moderate to moderately high blood pressure does not cause headache. However, headache may be associated with blood pressure that is very high and may be relieved if the blood pressure is reduced. The headache is usually at the back of the head, pulsating or throbbing in character, and is present on waking. Such headaches are rare in young people but increase in incidence in middle-aged and older people. Underlying causes for acute increased blood pressure should be sought and treated, e.g. phaeochromocytoma and pre-eclampsia.

1.26 Does sex cause headaches?

Headaches are sometimes linked to sexual activity and are known by a number of names:

- Benign sex headache
- Benign coital headache
- Orgasmic or coital cephalalgia
- Thunderclap headache.

The headache may occur pre- or postorgasm, in both cases lasting for several hours. Alternatively, the headache may occur at orgasm, when it is typically migrainous in character. The pain tends to start as orgasm is reached, as a dull cramping feeling at the back of the head. It increases in severity rapidly and is very intense for 5–15 minutes. It may then disappear or continue as a dull ache for up to 1 day.

Sufferers may experience regular attacks whenever they have intercourse, while the attacks may be unpredictable in others, separated by gaps of up to several years. The headaches are probably caused by muscle spasms in the neck.

While there is a certain amount of amusement associated with these headaches, they may severely affect the quality of life of sufferers, who are mostly young adults. Embarrassment may lead to sufferers being reluctant to talk about these headaches with their physicians.

HEADACHES AND LIFE STAGES

1.27 What headaches should be looked out for in children?

Children are prone to the common benign headaches of migraine, tension-type headache and chronic daily headache, although these conditions are less prevalent in children than in adults. Migraine may manifest with different symptoms in preadolescent children than in adults (*see* Q 1.11). However, by the time of adolescence, the symptoms are usually similar to those reported by adults. Most migraine sufferers have their first attacks during childhood and adolescence.

Other forms of childhood headache include:

- Headache associated with eye strain, usually in children requiring spectacles
- Headache associated with acute sinusitis or other infections
- In teenagers, some headaches may be related to alcohol or other recreational drug consumption

■ Headache following head or neck injury in a car accident.

1.28 What headaches should be looked out for in young and middle-aged adults?

Again, migraine, tension-type headache and chronic daily headache are common in young and middle-aged adults. Migraine achieves its peak prevalence at these ages. Cluster headache and short, sharp headaches may also occur.

Other forms of headache associated with this age group include:

■ Headache associated with eye strain, in middle-aged people as their eyesight alters
■ Headache associated with acute sinusitis or other infections
■ Headaches related to alcohol or other recreational drug consumption
■ Headaches related to the development of illnesses such as hypertension and prescribed drugs for certain conditions
■ Headache following head or neck injury in a car accident
■ Headaches related to sexual activity.

1.29 What headaches should be looked out for in older people?

Migraine prevalence decreases as people get older and migraine becomes relatively uncommon. However, tension-type headache and chronic daily headaches remain common.

Older people commonly have headaches associated with concomitant illnesses (e.g. hypertension) and concurrent medications.

Old age is associated with a range of severe, incapacitating headaches, including those due to:

■ Neuralgias: particularly trigeminal neuralgia and postherpetic neuralgia
■ Cranial arteritis
■ Temporomandibular joint dysfunction.

PQ PATIENT QUESTIONS

1.30 Does everybody get headaches?

Virtually everyone has had a headache at some time in their lives, even if it's just a hangover. However, a surprisingly large number of people get regular headaches. About three-quarters of people have one or more headaches every month.

1.31 What types of headache do people get?

Most headaches are benign and are not a cause of serious illnesses. The commonest headaches are migraine, tension-type headache and chronic daily headache, which, although painful, are not dangerous. Headaches may also be associated with eyestrain, taking too much alcohol or other drugs, and some illnesses. Meningitis and brain tumours are very rare causes of headache — there are always other features than the headache in these conditions. Older people are prone to some other painful types of headache that they should see their doctor about.

1.32 Who should I talk to about my headaches?

This really depends on how badly you are affected by your headaches. If the headache is not too bad and you can do your normal daily activities while you have the headache, you probably do not need to see your doctor. Your pharmacist should be able to give you the advice and treatment that you need.

However, if the headache stops you from doing your paid and household work, or stops you enjoying or taking part in leisure activities, you really should make an appointment to see your doctor to talk about it.

1.33 What is migraine?

Migraine is an illness that has several symptoms, including headache, sick feelings, sensitivity to light and sound, muscle pain and disrupted thought processes. The headache is usually one-sided and throbbing. Migraine occurs as a series of attacks lasting from a few hours to three days and sufferers are usually completely well between the attacks. Sufferers may have strange visual or other sensory symptoms (aura) before the headache that warn them that it is imminent. Migraine often runs in families and lasts for decades over the sufferer's life, usually from childhood or teens to late middle age.

1.34 What is tension-type headache?

Tension-type headache is usually a generalised headache that is dull and diffuse. It can last for a long time but generally does not prevent sufferers from conducting their normal activities. Feelings of nausea are not usually reported but sensitivity to light or sound may be present. This is the most common headache, with about half of all people having tension-type headache at least once a month.

1.35 What is chronic daily headache?

Chronic daily headache is any headache that occurs on more than half the days in each month. Any type of headache can be reported but the commonest types of chronic daily headache include chronic tension type headache and the combination of attacks of migraine and tension-type headache.

The commonest causes of chronic daily headache are head or neck injury (e.g. whiplash from a car accident) and overuse of painkilling medications (e.g. aspirin, paracetamol, codeine and ergotamine).

1.36 My 8-year old son is starting to get headaches. What is wrong?

There could be several causes of his headache but it is best to take him to your doctor to discover the true cause. He is almost certainly likely to have a benign headache that can be treated easily, probably tension-type headache, migraine or chronic daily headache. There may be other causes however:

■ If he gets headache when he reads, works on his computer or watches TV a lot, he may have eye strain. If so, spectacles will probably cure the headache.
■ If he has a fever and a discharge from his nose, he may have acute sinusitis. A course of antibiotics should clear this up.
■ If he has been in a car accident, he may have whiplash injuries.

1.37 My 14-year-old daughter has started to get bad headaches. What is wrong?

At her age, the most likely explanation is that she is developing migraine, which often starts during adolescence. This is even more likely if:

■ The headache is one-sided and throbbing.
■ She feels nauseous with the headache and can't stand bright lights and loud noises.
■ The headaches are associated with her menstrual periods.
■ One or more of her parents, grandparents, uncles or aunts have migraine.

You should take her to your doctor, who will be able to diagnose her headache and provide her with effective treatment.

1.38 I'm starting to get headaches every day. What is wrong with me?

You have developed the condition known as chronic daily headache. You may have had attacks of migraine or tension-type headache in the past, which have become more frequent over time. This increase in headache frequency may have occurred because:

■ You have been taking an increasing amount of painkillers recently.
■ You have suffered from a head or neck injury. This may be recent or could have occurred a long time ago, leading to chronic neck stiffness.

It is essential that you go to see your doctor for treatment, as the condition is unlikely to get better on its own. Some sufferers do find that stopping analgesics alone and regularising their lifestyles is enough to short circuit or break the cycle, but these are in the minority.

1.39 My mother, who is 68 years old, gets these awful headaches all the time. Each one lasts a few minutes but she gets several attacks every day. What is wrong?

Headaches such as these are quite common in older people, and could be due to a variety of causes. These conditions include trigeminal neuralgia and postherpetic neuralgia (after an attack of shingles). The important thing is to take her to see her doctor, who will be able to help with the pain.

Key clinical features of migraine

MIGRAINE AND OTHER HEADACHE TYPES

PATIENT QUESTIONS

DEFINITION OF MIGRAINE

2.1   How is migraine defined medically?

Migraine is defined as a common, painful condition of recurring headache attacks, commonly accompanied by nonheadache-associated symptoms. Attacks are sometimes preceded by aura symptoms. Attacks are classified as *migraine with aura* and *migraine without aura*, depending on the presence or absence of these symptoms. Migraine attacks last between 4 and 72 hours, with total freedom from symptoms between attacks. However, migraine is a heterogeneous disorder and attacks vary in their frequency, duration, severity and number of associated symptoms.

EPIDEMIOLOGY OF MIGRAINE

2.2   What is the incidence of migraine?

Migraine attacks usually start in childhood or adolescence; it is rare (but possible) for new cases to occur at over 30 years of age.

Several population studies have shown that the onset of migraine peaks in childhood and adolescence, then declines over time. Attacks tend to start at a younger age in boys than in girls. Also, attacks of migraine with aura tend to start at a younger age than attacks of migraine without aura. Onset of migraine after the age of 30 years is rare for both genders.

Physicians should look out for new cases of migraine with aura in boys aged 5 years upwards and girls aged 12 years and above. New cases of migraine without aura become frequent in boys aged 10 years upwards and girls aged 14 years and above.

2.3   What is the prevalence of migraine?

Migraine is a common disorder, mostly affecting young and middle-aged people, and is more common in women than in men.

Prevalence studies have been conducted primarily in Europe and North America and also in some Asian and African countries. The prevalence of migraine is remarkably constant around the world, with about 10–12% of the general adult population being affected. Assuming this, there are about 25 million migraine sufferers in the USA, eight million in Germany, six million each in France, Italy and the UK, and four million in Spain.

Migraine is also common in children. Overall, about 10% of children aged 5–15 years have migraine, rising from < 5% in those aged 5 years to 15% or more in those aged 12 years and older.

2.4   How common are the different subtypes of migraine?

Migraine without aura is much more common than migraine with aura, accounting for about 90% of patients. Most patients who have aura symptoms also suffer from attacks of migraine without aura. The idea, which may be prevalent in some patients, that a migraine attack has to have an associated aura, is therefore false. The majority of patients the physician sees with migraine will never have experienced an aura.

The rare migraine subtypes (*see Q 1.12*) are very uncommon, and the primary care physician may never see some of these forms during their careers.

2.5   Do gender and age affect the prevalence of migraine?

Migraine is two to three times more common in women than in men, presumed in part to be due to the influence of female hormones. However, peak prevalence occurs between the ages of 25 and 55 years for both genders.

Migraine is highly gender- and age-dependent. Overall, about 6% of men and 15% of women have migraine. In children, migraine prevalence increases with age for both genders but is more common in boys than in girls up to the age of 12 years. After this, migraine is much more common in girls and women than in boys and men.

In men, migraine prevalence increases gradually to about 8% at ages 30–40 years, then declines with age, until < 5% are affected at age >60 years

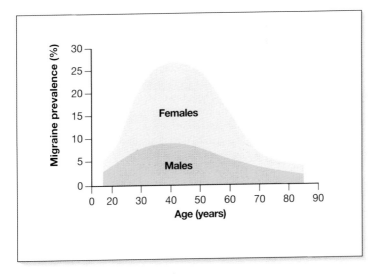

▲

Fig. 2.1 Prevalence of migraine. Reprinted from Staffa JA, Lipton RB, Stewart WF. *Rev Contemp Pharmacother* 1994;5:241–252 with permission from the Marius Press.

(*Fig. 2.1*). The pattern is slightly different in women. Migraine prevalence increases rapidly between the ages of 20 and 40 years, reaching a peak prevalence of over 25% between the ages of 40 and 45 years. Prevalence decreases thereafter, but is still common in women until about 65 years of age (*Fig. 2.1*). However, migraine becomes infrequent in elderly women, as well as men. Migraine with aura and migraine without aura are both more common in women than in men.

The reasons for the gender differences in migraine prevalence are not fully understood but are probably partly due to the influence of female hormones. Most women with migraine report attacks associated with their menses but also have attacks at other times during the menstrual cycle. Migraine attacks often improve or stop altogether during pregnancy, only to re-emerge after the birth of the child. The sudden decrease in plasma oestradiol that occurs during the onset of menstruation is implicated as a risk factor for migraine and may explain, in part, the female predominance of migraine. However, other factors must also be involved, as the gender difference in migraine prevalence persists after the menopause.

2.6 How does race affect the incidence and prevalence of migraine?

Migraine is common in all races but is more prevalent in white than in black or Asian races.

Historical studies in some African and Asian countries have generally indicated a lower prevalence of migraine in these countries than in Europe and North America. These results may have arisen from difficulties in conducting studies in third world countries, and studies conducted in more developed Far-Eastern Asian nations (e.g. Japan and Malaysia) showed prevalence rates similar to those reported for Western nations. However, racial, cultural and environmental differences may also contribute towards the low migraine prevalence reported in Africa and the Middle East.

A large survey conducted in the USA showed that migraine was more common in white Americans (20.4%) than in African (16.2%) and Asian Americans (9.2%) but was common in all three races. These results indicate that there may be race-related differences in vulnerability to migraine.

2.7 Do any other social or demographic factors affect the incidence and prevalence of migraine?

Although it is widely thought by patients and some physicians that migraine prevalence is related to social class, results from studies do not convincingly bear this out.

For many years it was believed that migraine was linked to high intelligence and social class. This was based on studies of patients attending physicians' clinics. More recent epidemiological studies have failed to show any such link – it seems likely that intelligence and social class predict the general tendency to consult a physician for care rather than any specific link to migraine.

Results from two studies in the USA indicated that migraine prevalence was inversely associated with the level of education and social class. However, numerous other studies conducted in the USA, Europe and Canada failed to show this association. The linkage of migraine to low social status is plausible. Poor living conditions, stress or lack of access to healthcare could lead to an increase in migraine prevalence. On the other hand, long-term exposure to migraine could lead to difficulties in work and career development, and a downward drift in social status. More evidence is required before such a link can be proven, however persuasive these arguments appear.

ASSOCIATION OF MIGRAINE WITH OTHER DISEASES

2.8   Is migraine associated with other diseases?

Although migraine is a self-limiting illness and resolves without sequelae, it leads to significant morbidity by itself and in combination with associated conditions. There is good evidence that migraine is linked to certain psychiatric disorders (particularly major depression, general anxiety, bipolar disorder and social phobia), epilepsy, stroke in women aged under 45 years and asthma. In the past, migraine has also been linked to chest pain, heart disease and angina, Raynaud's disease, bronchitis, gastrointestinal ulcers, irritable bowel syndrome, kidney disease, nose bleeds and urinary infections, although there is little evidence to substantiate these associations. Even so, the end result is that migraine sufferers experience the burden of associated illnesses as well as the migraine itself.

2.9   How is migraine associated with psychiatric disorders?

Migraine is strongly associated with major depression and major depression is likewise strongly associated with migraine. Each disorder increases the likelihood for the other. This linkage is not the same for depression and nonmigraine severe headaches. Here, nonmigraine headaches predict depression, but not vice versa.

Other work has demonstrated a link between migraine and somatostatin disorders, major depression, bipolar disorder and the anxiety disorders, general anxiety and social phobia. The combination of major depression and anxiety was particularly linked to migraine. There seems to be a distinct syndrome of anxiety in children, which is followed by migraine and episodes of depression in adults.

Migraine is also linked to certain personality disorders, especially neuroticism, which is particularly prevalent in patients who are prone to tension-type headaches as well as migraine.

The physician treating patients with migraine should be aware of the possibility of these co-morbid psychiatric illnesses. Also, patients with depression should be investigated to see if any associated headaches are due to migraine.

2.10 How is migraine associated with stroke?

There has been much interest in the postulated link between migraine and stroke. In the Physician's Health Study, the risk of stroke in migraine sufferers was about two-fold higher than that in people without migraine, especially in those who had migraine with aura.

Several specific studies have shown that the risk of ischaemic (but not haemorrhagic) stroke was increased in women aged under 35 or 45 years old who had migraine with or without aura, and was exacerbated by oral contraceptive use, smoking and high blood pressure. There was no link between migraine and stroke for any other patient group.

The originally reported link between migraine and stroke is therefore probably coincidental, due to coexisting migraine and stroke and stroke that exhibits clinical features of migraine. Headache is a common feature of stroke and may be confused with a migraine attack. True migraine-induced stroke (migrainous infarction [see Q 3.8]) is very rare and is restricted to young women. The physician should advise young female migraine sufferers not to smoke and to use a contraceptive pill with a low oestrogen dose, if they require this form of contraception. Their blood pressure should also be checked. Patients with prolonged aura symptoms may need to be checked for the possibility of transient ischaemic attack (TIA), reversible ischaemic neurological deficit (RIND) or cerebral infarction, depending on the duration of the symptoms (see Q 1.12).

2.11 How is migraine linked with epilepsy?

There is about a 2.4-fold higher risk of migraine in patients and their relatives who have epilepsy compared with relatives who do not have epilepsy. There is therefore a strong association between migraine and epilepsy, which is independent of seizure type, aetiology, age at onset or family history of epilepsy. It has been proposed that there is a state of underlying neuronal hyperexcitability that increases the risk for both disorders.

The relationship between migraine and epilepsy is complex. Seizures may occur during attacks of migraine without aura, where the condition has sometimes been known as migralepsy. In other cases, seizures with visual symptoms analogous to, but quite different from, symptoms of the migraine aura may be accompanied or followed by headaches that are similar or identical to migraine (the 'ictal' headaches). In these cases, the seizure probably triggers migraine by activating trigeminovascular or brainstem mechanisms (*see Q 2.41*). It is important that the physician is able to distinguish the visual seizure symptoms from those of migraine aura in these cases (*see Q 3.9*).

2.12   How is migraine linked with asthma?

There seems to be a genetic link between migraine and asthma. Asthma is more frequently reported in children of mothers with migraine than in those of mothers without migraine. The mechanism of this link is unknown at present but the physician should suspect migraine as the source of headache in children whose mothers are asthma sufferers. In addition, certain asthma medications show promise for the treatment of migraine (*see Q 8.12*).

THE NATURAL HISTORY OF THE MIGRAINE ATTACK

2.13   How does the migraine attack develop?

The migraine attack involves a cascade of neurological, psychological and physical changes that generally occur in a predictable manner. Clinically,

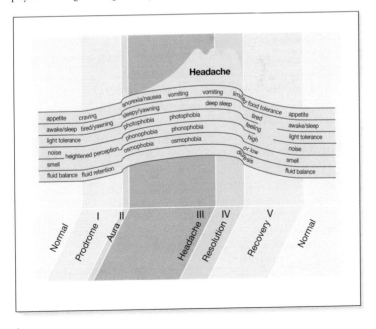

Fig. 2.2 The five phases of the migraine attack: prodrome, aura, headache, resolution and recovery.

the acute attack is divided into five phases that occur in series: *prodrome, aura, headache, resolution* and *recovery* (*Fig. 2.2*).

2.14 What are the features of the migraine prodrome?

The preheadache prodrome phase is characterised by nonspecific symptoms such as:

- ■ Tiredness and yawning
- ■ Mood disruption
- ■ Muscle pain
- ■ Food cravings
- ■ Heightened perception
- ■ Fluid retention.

Prodrome symptoms occur before about 50–70% of migraine attacks and last for several hours to several days. Patients may not be aware of the significance of these symptoms unless educated about them. However, the majority of migraine sufferers can predict at least some of their migraine attacks from these symptoms. Some of the symptoms, e.g. muscle tension, food cravings and heightened sensory awareness, may be mistaken for migraine *triggers* (*see Q 2.46*) by the patient. Prodrome symptoms arise presumably due to neurochemical disruption. They often continue throughout the attack but are overshadowed by the headache phase.

2.15 What are the features of the migraine aura?

Only about 10% of migraine sufferers experience aura symptoms – and not in all their attacks. Aura symptoms are reversible, localised neurological symptoms that are variable in timing and symptomatology. These symptoms typically occur at the end of the prodrome, last up to 1 hour, usually immediately precede the onset of headache and may include:

- ■ Visual disturbances (temporary blind spots, blurred vision, scotomas or a pattern of flashing lights or zigzag lines)
- ■ Speech disturbances such as word-salading
- ■ Sensations affecting other areas of the body, such as tingling, dizziness, numbness, sensory loss and limb weakness.

However, aura symptoms can also occur on their own without headache sequelae, can overlap with the prodrome and headache, or there can be a gap between the prodrome and aura. The presence of aura symptoms is not predictive of the severity of the following headache. Attacks of migraine without aura may be as, or more, severe than those of migraine with aura. Auras are believed to occur due to electrical events initiated by a wave of spreading cortical depression in the brain (*see Q 2.40*).

2.16 What are the features of the headache phase of the migraine attack?

The headache phase of migraine is characterised by headache that usually starts with mild (dull, diffuse) pain but which can escalate to moderate or severe disabling pain that leads to disruption of the sufferer's normal activities.

> ## Symptoms of the headache phase
> The following symptoms are typically reported:
> - *Headache* – the most prominent feature, which is usually throbbing, unilateral, aggravated by activity and moderate to very severe in intensity.
> - *Photophobia and phonophobia*, reported by the majority of sufferers, which may cause them to have to lie down in a darkened room until the attack ends.
> - *Nausea*, reported by half or more of sufferers.
> - *Vomiting*, reported by 20% or less of sufferers, but indicative of a particularly severe attack.
> - Other symptoms suggesting autonomic activation are also seen, such as nasal congestion, rhinorrhoea, lacrimation, and diarrhoea.

2.17 What are the features of the resolution phase of the migraine attack?

After the headache peaks in intensity, it may gradually lessen and disappear over a period of hours. Sometimes, however, resolution may be triggered by a bout of vomiting, or sufferers may settle into a period of deep sleep and wake up with the symptoms resolved.

2.18 What are the features of the recovery phase of the migraine attack?

The final postheadache recovery phase is characterised by lingering symptoms, much like a hangover without the headache. These include:

- Gastrointestinal symptoms with a sick, queasy stomach and food intolerance
- Decreased concentration and occasional cognitive difficulties
- Sore muscles
- An overall sense of fatigue.

These symptoms can lead to disruption to the sufferer's normal activities, similar to a hangover (they are often called the 'migraine hangover'). In contrast, some sufferers experience euphoria and a sense of wellbeing. The recovery phase can last from several hours to 48 hours.

2.19 **How do menstrual migraine attacks differ from nonmenstrual attacks?**

Menstrual migraine is defined solely by its timing within the menstrual cycle. This can be an arbitrary definition but most studies now use a time window of day −1 to +3 of the menstrual period. Any other migraine attacks are nonmenstrual by this definition.

Menstrual migraine attacks have been thought for a long time to be more severe and more difficult to treat than nonmenstrual attacks. However, the evidence for this is slim and more recent studies indicate that there is probably little difference between the two types of attack.

The physician should view menstrual migraine attacks as part of the spectrum of headaches experienced by that sufferer. Very few women will have solely menstrual migraine attacks. The management strategies used for menstrual migraine attacks can generally be the same as those used for nonmenstrual attacks (*see* Q 5.70).

2.20 **Does an understanding of the natural history of migraine influence the treatment that can be given?**

In practice, most migraine attacks are treated during the headache phase, by which time the patient can be certain that they are suffering from a migraine attack. However, it is of obvious advantage if migraine can be treated earlier than this, during the prodrome or aura. Treatment during these phases has the potential to abolish the headache altogether or reduce its intensity. Many patients can recognise prodrome symptoms and the aura is usually obvious, so treatment is feasible for many patients during these phases. Wherever possible, the physician should recommend that the migraine patient treats the migraine before the headache develops (*see* Q 5.41). However, treatment with the triptans should be reserved until the headache phase has developed (*see* Q 5.44).

The resolution and recovery phases of the migraine attack may be lengthy and distressing for the patient. It may also be appropriate, therefore, to provide therapy for the patient who is unable to function normally during these phases (*see* Q 8.5).

BURDEN OF MIGRAINE TO THE SUFFERER

2.21 **What do we mean by the burden of migraine?**

Migraine is a heterogeneous disorder characterised by attacks that vary in frequency, duration, severity and symptomatology. This variability exists both between different sufferers and within the individual sufferer over their separate attacks. Migraine sufferers experience disability and reduced quality of life during their attacks, which, over a lifetime's illness, can lead to profound consequences on their work, family and leisure lifestyles. This forms the personal burden of migraine, experienced by the sufferer and their family and friends.

There is also a financial burden of migraine that is borne by society in general – the societal burden. The costs of treating migraine in the medical setting form the direct costs, while the costs of lost work time due to absence and reduced productivity form the indirect costs (*see Q 2.32*).

2.22 How frequently do migraine attacks occur?

The frequency of migraine attacks is highly variable, both between different patients, and in separate attacks for the individual sufferer. The average frequency is about 1–2 attacks per month but may vary from < 1 to > 50 attacks per year.

2.23 How long do migraine attacks last?

The duration of migraine attacks is also highly variable between different patients and between different attacks in the individual patient. The average duration is about 24 hours but varies from < 4 hours to 3 days. The International Headache Society diagnostic criteria for migraine state that the attack should last a minimum of 4 hours but in practice some patients have attacks that last as little as 2 hours.

2.24 What are the main symptoms of migraine that are burdensome?

The main symptom of migraine is a headache that is usually moderate to severe in intensity, throbbing and one-sided. This is usually accompanied by photophobia and/or phonophobia and nausea, and lethargy may also be common. Vomiting is relatively infrequent.

The pain of the migraine headache is the most important symptom to the migraine patient and is the main reason given for seeking medical care. However, pain is subjective; some patients may be incapacitated by a relatively moderate headache, while others can operate normally even when the headache is very severe.

Symptoms associated with the headache of migraine may be equally, or more important to the patient as the headache. Nausea, photophobia and phonophobia can all cause patients distress and prevent them from conducting their normal activities. Vomiting, when it occurs, is particularly disabling.

Migraine therefore consists of a constellation of symptoms that vary in incidence, severity and duration between attacks. This grouping of symptoms undoubtedly contributes to the severity of migraine as perceived by the patient, e.g. the combination of severe headache with nausea and photophobia having far more impact than any of the individual symptoms on their own.

Prodrome and aura, when they occur, can be frightening, as patients may become worried about the upcoming attack. Symptoms during the recovery phase may also be distressing, especially if the patient is recovering from a severe attack.

2.25 Does migraine affect the quality of life of sufferers?

The quality of life (QOL) of migraine sufferers during their attacks is significantly poorer than that of the general healthy population, especially with respect to pain and interference to their daily and social lives. The QOL also decreases as the severity of the migraine increases.

The QOL of migraine sufferers is also poorer than QOL in other chronic diseases that are usually considered to be more serious than migraine, such as hypertension, depression, osteoarthritis and type II diabetes (*Fig. 2.3*). Migraine sufferers reported significantly more pain and restrictions to their daily activities than people with all these other diseases. They also reported significantly poorer mental health and social functioning than all groups except for those people with depression.

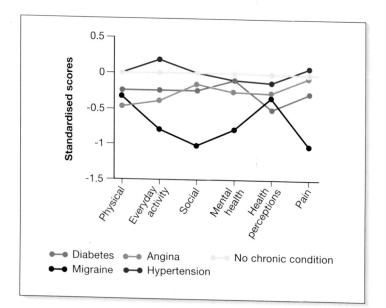

Fig. 2.3 Quality of life of migraine sufferers compared to those suffering from other chronic diseases.

Moreover, migraine sufferers experience suboptimal QOL even when they are symptom-free between attacks. Compared to a control group, migraine sufferers reported disturbed contentment, vitality and sleep, more subjective symptoms and a reduced sense of wellbeing. Emotional distress, anxiety and sex lives were all worse in the group of migraine sufferers.

2.26   Does migraine cause disability?

Migraine is a remarkably disabling condition, with most sufferers reporting significant impact associated with their attacks in all areas of their lifestyles. Migraine-related disability can be considered as the objective effects of the illness on sufferers' lifestyles, including their work and leisure activities, rather than subjective effects expressed as symptoms and QOL. Disability is defined by the World Health Organization as 'a restriction or lack (resulting from an impairment) of ability to perform an activity in the manner or within the range considered normal for a human being'.

Studies from around the world have shown that migraine causes significant disability in its sufferers, with two-thirds or more reporting at least mild disability and a third or more reporting moderate to severe disability (*Fig. 2.4*). In a UK study, two-thirds of migraine sufferers reported that migraine disrupted their lives, with three-quarters having to lie down during attacks (*Table 2.1*). A second study indicated that between one-third and two-thirds of migraine sufferers in the UK (an estimated 1.9–3.8 million people) felt that they were not in control of their migraine and the way it affected their day-to-day lives.

The consequences of migraine-related disability are seen in patients' lifestyles, including employment, unpaid work and family and leisure activities.

2.27   How does migraine affect the employment of working sufferers?

Migraine attacks cause a considerable amount of lost time from work for sufferers, and may even lead to unemployment in severe cases.

In a study conducted in the USA, each working migraine sufferer missed an average of 4.4 days of work per year and the equivalent of 12 further days due to reduced productivity during attacks. In the UK, half of sufferers reported missing work and over two-thirds reported difficulty performing work during attacks (*Table 2.1*). Migraine may even lead to unemployment. In a primary care organisation in the USA, the unemployment rate was 2–4-fold higher in severely affected migraine sufferers than in the general population.

In general, migraine sufferers do try to go to work during their attacks but are unable to work at their normal productivity level.

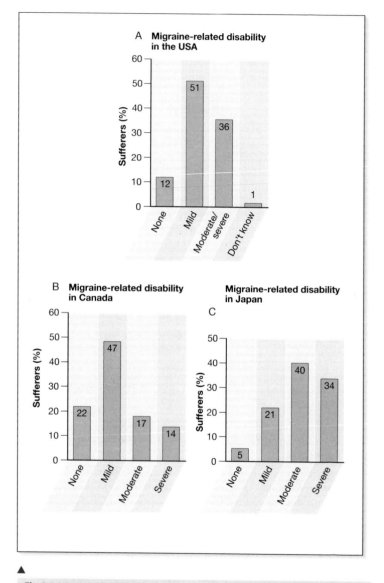

Fig. 2.4 Migraine-related disability reported in studies conducted in the USA (a), Canada (b) and Japan (c).

TABLE 2.1 Impact of migraine on sufferers' lifestyles in the UK	
Disability	Proportion of sufferers (%)
Physical functioning	
Always have to lie down	76
Not in control of life	34
Disruption of life	67
Employment	
Usually miss work	50
Difficulty performing work	72
Cancel appointments/meetings	67
Rely on other people	45
Perceived effect on promotion	15
Unpaid work	
Postpone household chores	90
Family and leisure activities	
Relations with family and friends affected	54

2.28 How does migraine affect students' education?

School and college work can be severely affected in young migraine sufferers. In a Scottish study, children with migraine were absent from school from all causes for significantly longer periods than those without migraine (7.8 days versus 3.7 days per year, $P < 0.0001$).

2.29 How does migraine affect unpaid work?

Migraine has a profound effect on sufferers' ability to do unpaid work such as housework, shopping and looking after children and other dependants. In a UK study, 90% of migraine sufferers reported that they postponed their household work during an attack (*Table 2.1*).

Unpaid work is particularly badly affected during migraine attacks. If sufferers have to give up one activity during their migraines, it is usually this one.

2.30 How does migraine affect family and leisure activities?

Several studies around the world have shown that migraine attacks commonly result in the cancellation of social events and affect relationships with partners, children, friends and other people.

Several studies from Canada, the UK and the USA have shown that up to 50% or more of sufferers report that migraine leads to the cancellation of family and social activities. However, the effects may be more insidious. Many migraine sufferers report that their attacks cause tension between them and their partners and may even impair their sexual relationships. The impact on children is also considerable. The vast majority of migraine sufferers report that their attacks interfere with their relationships with their children, and the end result is often the child exhibiting attention-seeking or hostile behaviour.

Not just family relationships are upset by migraine. A third or more of migraine sufferers state that the condition affects their relationships with friends and other people.

2.31 Are there any long-term disease consequences associated with migraine?

Anxiety, depression and fear are common among migraine sufferers, either as a direct result of the condition or due to coexisting psychiatric disorders. Sufferers are often unwilling to go to parties or other social situations due to the fear that these will trigger an attack.

In the long term, feelings of guilt, helplessness and despair can occur when sufferers see no end to the illness or think no effective treatment is available. There are many anecdotal accounts from sufferers of people losing their jobs and being divorced as a direct result of their migraine.

BURDEN OF MIGRAINE ON SOCIETY

2.32 What do we mean by the direct and indirect cost of an illness?

The personal burden of migraine is reflected in an economic burden on society. This economic burden is assessed by calculating direct and indirect costs.

Direct costs place values on resources allocated to the diagnosis, treatment and rehabilitation of patients with the illness. These comprise:

- Consultations with primary care physicians, specialists and alternative practitioners
- Tests, hospitalisations and care in casualty/emergency room departments
- Prescription and over-the-counter drugs.

Indirect costs estimate the value of lost productivity due to mortality and morbidity, including lost earnings, reduced productivity and outputs, losses in education and job promotion, and unwanted job changes. Most indirect costs for migraine are due to work absence and reduced work productivity.

2.33 What are the direct medical costs of migraine?

Most migraine sufferers consult a primary care physician at some time, although in Europe consultation with a specialist is infrequent and hospitalisations and emergency room consultations are rare. In North America and some European countries, many sufferers see alternative practitioners for their migraine. Most migraine sufferers rely on over-the-counter medications for therapy.

The end result is that direct costs for migraine are relatively low, estimated at about $15 million to $1 billion annually in Western countries. The total annual costs of medical care in 1993 (adjusted to $US) were:

- USA = $1 billion
- Sweden = $13 million
- UK = $45 million
- Netherlands = $300 million
- Australia = $31 million.

Direct costs of migraine are therefore relatively low. However, they are rising, partly due to the introduction of new drugs such as the triptans. At present, total direct costs of migraine in the USA exceed $2 billion annually.

2.34   What are the indirect costs of migraine?

Indirect costs of an illness estimate the total days lost from paid work due to sickness absence and lost productivity, then calculating the resulting income lost due to this lost time. Indirect costs are very large for migraine, being estimated as equivalent to about $0.5–13 billion per year in large Western countries. The total annual indirect costs of migraine due to lost productivity in 1993 (adjusted to US$) were:

- USA = $13 billion
- Sweden = $1.6 billion
- UK = $1.1–1.3 billion
- Netherlands = $1.2 billion
- Spain = $1.1 billion
- Australia = $568 million.

Indirect costs therefore provide the main economic burden of migraine. They could be reduced if new effective treatments reduced the amount of work time lost due to migraine. A cost benefit to society would result if the increased direct costs from a new therapy were less than the savings in indirect costs obtained through increased work productivity.

2.35   Does migraine impose a societal burden that cannot be measured in financial terms?

Much of the burden of migraine cannot be captured in economic terms. Economists describe such factors as pain, suffering and reduced QOL in sufferers and their families, caregivers and co-workers as 'intangibles', which cannot be valued using economic analyses. However, they are no less important for this and form the main part of the personal burden of migraine (see Q 2.21).

PATHOGENESIS OF MIGRAINE

2.36 What are the overall causative factors associated with migraine?

The underlying causes of migraine have only recently been elucidated and are still not completely understood. Genetic, central, vascular and neural components are all involved. Certain biochemical and physiological risk factors are hypothesised to predispose sufferers to migraine. Finally,

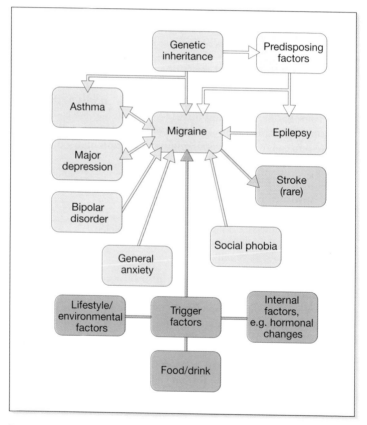

Fig. 2.5 Overview of the relationship between migraine and genetic, predisposing and precipitating factors, and concurrent diseases.

many precipitating *trigger* factors are proposed to initiate specific attacks. *Figure 2.5* illustrates the interactions between these causative factors.

2.37   What is the evidence for migraine being an inherited illness?

Migraine has long been observed to 'run in families', which gave impetus to investigations into the genetic nature of the disease. However, inheritance of migraine is complex. Migraine with aura seems to be determined by genetic factors, whilst migraine without aura is determined by a combination of genetic and environmental factors.

Inheritance of migraine is multifactorial through several genes. Recent evidence (albeit indirect from studies on familial hemiplegic migraine) has implicated a mutation in the gene for the voltage-dependent calcium ion channel protein on chromosome 19 in migraine, as well as in other episodic and chronic neurological disorders (*Fig. 2.6*). This indicates that migraine may be a form of channelopathy. However, other genes are involved, including a locus on chromosome 1.

2.38   What do we mean by calling migraine a 'channelopathy'?

Channelopathy disorders (e.g. the ataxias) share several features that are seen in migraine:

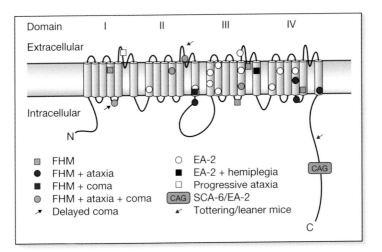

Fig. 2.6 Different missense mutations in the calcium ion channel genes in different phenotypes of familial hemiplegic migraine (FHM) and related channelopathies. EA-2 = episodic ataxia type 2; SCA-6 = spinocerebellar ataxia type 6. Reprinted from Kors EE, Terwindt GM, Vermeulen FL et al. Ann Neurol 2001;49:753–760 with permission.

- Episodic manifestations with variable frequency and duration of attacks
- Spontaneous remission of attacks
- Onset in the early decades of life and reduction in prevalence in later life
- Identifiable triggers for attacks such as exercise, hormones, stress and food.

Mutations of the calcium channel gene may be implicated in the channelopathies (*Fig. 2.6*). If the calcium channel defect is a basic abnormality in migraine, it may result in a defective release of neurotransmitters and altered brain and energy metabolism, both of which lead to a state of central neuronal hyperexcitability. This is thought to be a fundamental abnormality in migraine.

2.39 What is the evidence for a 'migraine generator' in the brain?

Brainstem nuclei and periaqueductal grey matter (PAG) have been implicated in the generation of migraine. These are components of ascending and descending pain pathways. Positron emission tomography studies have shown that there is activation of the brainstem and areas of the cerebral cortex during spontaneous migraine attacks, with a resultant increased blood flow in these areas. Cerebral blood flow changes do not cause the pain of migraine. This is due to the subsequent activation of the trigeminal vascular system (*see Q 2.42*). However, activation of sites in the brainstem seems to be the first change to take place in the brain during a migraine attack – these sites are hence known as the 'migraine generator'.

2.40 What is the current understanding for how aura develops?

Clinical, imaging and blood flow studies clearly indicate that the migraine aura originates from the cerebral cortex. The visual aura spreads laterally in one hemisphere, spreading at a steady speed, and accelerating and enlarging as it spreads. Nonvisual aura symptoms also spread at a slow pace and, if there is more than one type of aura symptom, they occur in sequence.

Several theories have been put forward to explain the migraine aura, including arterial spasm and ischaemia. However, the only known disturbance that explains these features is Leao's cortical spreading depression (CSD). This involves a slowly spreading cortical hypoperfusion, followed by hyperaemia in many cases. Blood flow in the cerebral hemispheres is normal in attacks of migraine without aura, indicating that the migraine aura and headache are caused by two separate mechanisms. However, CSD may also lead to pain through activation of the trigeminal vascular system.

2.41 What is the neurovascular theory of migraine pathogenesis?

Two separate hypotheses have been proposed for explaining the pathogenesis of migraine – the vascular and the neural theories:

■ The vascular theory proposes that migraine is caused by abnormal dilatation of cerebral vessels, possibly caused by decreased concentrations of blood 5-hydroxytryptamine (5-HT).
■ The neural theory proposes that inflammatory mechanisms in the brainstem are responsible for initiating a migraine attack.

These two theories have now been combined into the neurovascular hypothesis, which incorporates components from both theories and in which 5-HT plays a major role (*Fig. 2.7*):

1. When a susceptible nervous system confronts a migraine-provoking environment, neurochemical changes occur, often resulting in premonitory symptoms. Eventually a critical threshold is reached and an area in the brainstem is activated (the hypothesised 'migraine generator').
2. Increases in regional cerebral blood flow result, slightly opposite to the headache side.
3. This stimulates sympathetic neurons and brainstem 5-HT- and noradrenaline-containing neurons to induce dilatation in intracranial blood vessels such as those in the meninges and large cerebral arteries.
4. These arteries are pain sensitive through a large innervation through sensory nerves in the trigeminal ganglion.
5. Activation of these sensory nerves causes the release of the inflammatory mediators substance P and calcitonin gene-related peptide (CGRP), which produce inflammation and distension of the vessel.
6. These stimuli produce pain signals that are transmitted centrally via the trigeminal nerve.

2.42 How do the pain and other symptoms of the migraine attack develop?

Migraine is an idiopathic pain (i.e. with no tissue injury or detectable pathology) and all the main migraine symptoms may result from activation of the trigeminal vascular system.

Vasodilatation and neural inflammation rapidly sensitise the first-order trigeminal nerve, resulting in a throbbing head pain that is aggravated by non-nociceptive stimuli, such as arterial pulsations and activities that increase intracranial pressure, including physical exercise, bending down, coughing and sneezing. This mechanism explains why the migraine headache is exacerbated by physical activity and why the sufferer usually prefers to lie down and stay quiet during their attacks.

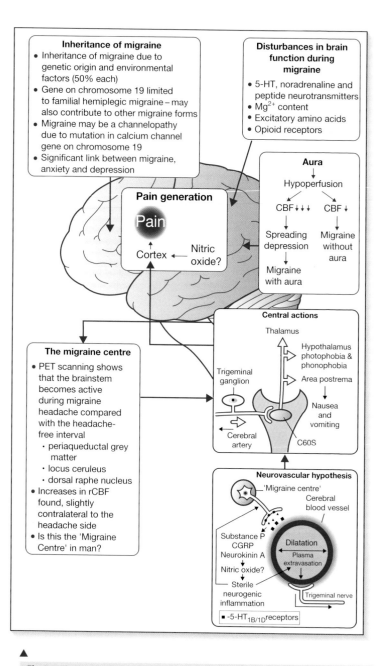

Fig. 2.7 The neurovascular theory of migraine pathogenesis.

Activated first-order neurons transmit pain to the second-order neurons in the trigeminal nuclei. These latter neurons in turn are connected to other important brainstem centres, particularly the nausea and vomiting centres. This mechanism explains the incidence of nausea and vomiting during migraine attacks, triggered by 5-HT release within the vomiting centre of the brain.

Further activation of the trigeminal system involves third-order neurons from the thalamus to the cortex, resulting in the migraine symptoms of photophobia, phonophobia, osmophobia and allodynia (non-nociceptive stimuli producing pain and discomfort).

Other migraine symptoms that may occur, including difficulties in concentration and impairment of cognitive functions, may arise from disturbances in brainstem centres responsible for attention.

2.43 How do female reproductive hormones contribute towards migraine development?

The dynamics of oestrogen metabolism has a key role in migraine. The primary trigger of menstrual migraine seems to be the rapid withdrawal of oestrogen, rather than sustained high or low oestrogen levels. Also, sustained high levels of oestrogen associated with pregnancy and sustained low levels associated with the menopause can be associated with the reduction or disappearance of migraine attacks.

The menstrual cycle involves a sequence of interactions between the hypothalamus, pituitary, ovaries and endometrium. Oestrogen and progestins have potent effects on central serotonergic and opioid neurons, altering their activity and density. It is likely that the relationship of oestrogen to migraine is modulated through these neurons. The mechanism of how this occurs is unknown, but may be via a nitric-oxide dependent system (see Q 2.44).

2.44 Is there a single biochemical 'trigger' for migraine?

Nitric oxide (NO) seems to be an important trigger for the induction of primary headaches. The administration of glycerol trinitrate (an NO donor) induces migraine, cluster headache and tension-type headache in susceptible patients. It has been hypothesised that the release of NO from blood vessels, perivascular nerve endings or brain tissue is a molecular mechanism that triggers the symptoms of spontaneous migraine attacks. Inhibitors of the enzyme that synthesises NO (NO synthase) are now being evaluated as acute treatments for migraine attacks (see Q 8.10).

2.45 Are there any biochemical factors that are implicated in migraine pathogenesis?

Research has shown that migraine sufferers can have certain metabolic abnormalities that have been hypothesised to predispose them to migraine. The factors identified so far include:

- Changes to platelet structure and function
- Dysfunction and instability in the autonomic nervous system
- Abnormal function of the opiate receptor
- Changes in ovarian hormone levels
- Decreased levels of metabolic enzymes
- Electroencephalographic (EEG) abnormalities.

However, the relevance of these abnormalities to migraine pathogenesis is not clear. Without further evidence, the coexistence of migraine and these putative risk factors may be purely coincidental. Alternatively, these abnormalities may arise as an effect of repeated migraine attacks rather than be a cause of them.

MIGRAINE TRIGGER FACTORS

2.46 What do we mean by migraine trigger factors?

Most migraine attacks occur spontaneously. However, some internal and/or external stimuli are implicated in the precipitation of certain attacks, as they precede the attack by a short interval. These are known as trigger factors.

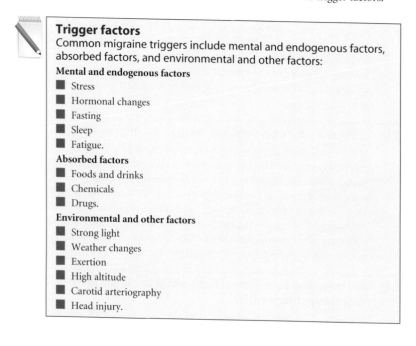

Trigger factors

Common migraine triggers include mental and endogenous factors, absorbed factors, and environmental and other factors:

Mental and endogenous factors

- Stress
- Hormonal changes
- Fasting
- Sleep
- Fatigue.

Absorbed factors

- Foods and drinks
- Chemicals
- Drugs.

Environmental and other factors

- Strong light
- Weather changes
- Exertion
- High altitude
- Carotid arteriography
- Head injury.

2.47   Do stress and lifestyle choices cause migraine attacks?

Stress is strongly linked with migraine attacks. Anxiety, tension, excitement, depression, shock and frustration may all lead to migraine attacks. Some migraine sufferers always report attacks when they are severely stressed, e.g. when they have to make a presentation or take part in an important meeting at work. Interestingly, the cessation of stress can also lead to attacks. Migraine attacks are often reported not during the working week when the sufferer is stressed, but at the weekend, when they are more rested (although lifestyle changes may also play a role here, see below). There is a clear link between migraine and psychiatric disorders (*see Q 2.9*), which may explain in part the link between migraine and stress.

Migraine may also be triggered by missed or irregular meals, sleeping too little or too much and fatigue. All of these factors may be related to the effects of stress. These lifestyle changes also tend to occur when migraine sufferers change their lifestyles at weekends and holidays, sleeping longer, having a different pattern of meals and eating different things than they do in the working week.

Stress may possibly lead to migraine by inducing the state of central neuronal hyperexcitability that seems to be present in all migraine sufferers.

2.48   Which foods and drinks may cause migraine attacks?

Numerous foods and drinks have been implicated as triggers for migraine attacks. Among the commonest are:

- Chocolate
- Cheese and other dairy products
- Fruit
- Alcoholic drinks (particularly red wine)
- Fried fatty foods
- Vegetables
- Tea and coffee
- Wheat
- Seafood.

Sufferers typically report that the consumption of these foodstuffs shortly precedes the migraine attacks. Many believe that they are a direct cause of the attack. Some foodstuffs may contain chemicals that can induce the migraine attack, e.g. red wine contains vasodilators that act via a NO-mediated pathway.

2.49   Which chemicals and drugs cause migraine attacks?

Chemicals implicated as migraine triggers include sodium nitrite, tartrazine and benzoic acid. Many patients also report that exposure to strong smells associated with chemicals such as perfume, paint and petrol can precede their attacks.

Many drugs are implicated as migraine triggers, including oestrogen, ergotamine (in overuse or withdrawal), indomethacin, nifedipine, dipyridamole and reserpine.

2.50 Which environmental factors cause migraine attacks?

Patients report that several environmental factors can lead to migraine. Changes in the weather, excessive heat, light or noise, exertion and high altitude are all reported to trigger attacks. As with stress, these factors could induce the state of central neuronal hyperexcitability that is implicated in migraine.

2.51 What other migraine triggers are there?

Migraine may follow carotid arteriography and head injury. Head injury often causes headache and is a risk factor for chronic daily headache (see Q 1.19). Migraine is also closely associated with female hormones. Attacks often first occur at puberty and are associated with menstruation and the use of oral contraceptives. The pattern of migraine often alters during pregnancy or the menopause (see Qs 5.71, 5.72).

2.52 Do migraine triggers really exist or are there other explanations for these associations?

Trigger factors are certainly involved in the development of migraine attacks but the physician should be sceptical when a patient states that a specific factor always triggers their attacks. The quality of the evidence for migraine triggers is poor, with most studies simply involving the collation of patient reports.

Of the proposed trigger factors described above, there is reasonable evidence and/or a plausible case for believing that the following factors may cause migraine attacks:

- Stress
- Hormonal changes in women
- Red wine
- Head injury.

The risk of developing migraine is increased if more than one trigger factor is present, e.g. if the sufferer is stressed and tries to relax with a glass of red wine.

While trigger factors certainly play a role in the genesis of some patients' attacks, there is often little objective evidence to substantiate their general prevalence. The simple coexistence of the putative trigger factor and a migraine attack does not necessarily mean there is a causal relationship between the two. For example, there are no good quality studies to substantiate the belief that most foodstuffs can induce migraine attacks. An alternative explanation is that in the prodrome phase of the migraine attack, sufferers sometimes have cravings for certain foods or drinks (*see Q 2.14*). These may then be blamed for causing the attacks, when they are in fact a consequence of them.

MIGRAINE AND OTHER HEADACHE TYPES

2.53   What are the relationships between migraine and chronic daily headache?

Migraine can be confused with chronic daily headache in clinical practice. Patients experiencing very frequent headaches (present on > 15 days of each month) that last for more than 4 hours are unlikely to have migraine alone but probably have chronic daily headache. Chronic daily headache is relatively common, affecting about 5% of the population. The condition may arise as migraine or episodic tension-type headache, which subsequently becomes altered in character due to:

■ Overuse of analgesics or ergotamine preparations taken for a primary headache disorder – there is the potential for the development of a 'spiral' of increasing headache frequency, analgesic overuse, development of rebound headaches and eventually chronic headache
■ A head or neck injury occurring at any time in the sufferer's lifetime.

The typical clinical picture is one of episodic migraine symptoms superimposed on a background of tension-type headache symptoms, although chronic tension-type headaches and chronic migraines can occur on their own (*see Q 1.18*). The management of CDH is different from that of migraine (*see Q 6.6*).

2.54   What are the relationships between migraine and tension-type headache?

Migraine is essentially a different disorder from tension-type headache. The majority of the general population experience tension-type headaches but never have migraine. As would be expected, migraine sufferers also commonly have tension-type headaches and migraine may aggravate and precipitate tension-type headaches. However, migraine sufferers experience a spectrum of headache, including 'pure' migraine, 'pure' tension-type headaches and headaches that seem to be a mixture of the two headache types (*see Q 3.12*). All of these headaches seem to be manifestations of the migraine process and can be treated by migraine-specific medications. Presumably, all these headaches result from the convergence of various peripheral inputs into the trigeminal vascular system.

2.55 What are the relationships between migraine and other headaches?

The symptoms of migraine may be confused by patients and physicians with those of several other headache disorders, including cluster headache, short, sharp headaches, sinus headaches and other forms of facial pain, and secondary (sinister) headaches. However, these headaches are quite different from migraine. In practice, it is a relatively simple job for the physician to differentiate between migraine and other headache types (*see Q 3.7*).

PQ PATIENT QUESTIONS

2.56 Who gets migraine?

Migraine is quite common, affecting about one in 20 men and one in five women. It usually starts in childhood or adolescence and is most common in young and middle-aged adults. Migraine often stops as people get older. All types of people can get migraine, although it is more common in white people than in black or Asian people. The old fashioned idea that migraine is linked to high intelligence is a fallacy. Anyone can get migraine, irrespective of their social class.

2.57 Is migraine linked to other diseases?

The majority of migraine sufferers have no other illnesses, are completely well between their attacks and lead normal lives. Migraine sufferers should not be stigmatised into the sick role or treated as if they are disabled. However, migraine sufferers do have a higher risk than normal of having certain other diseases. Chief among these are some psychiatric disorders, mainly depression, anxiety, bipolar disorder and social phobia. They may also be prone to epilepsy and asthma. On the other hand, there is no real extra risk of stroke in migraine patients, even in those who experience aura.

2.58 How can I tell if a migraine attack is on the way?

Not everyone can tell if they are going to get a migraine attack and many attacks arrive without warning. However, some people do get warning symptoms in the hours before the attack starts properly. It is worth looking out for signs such as mood changes (e.g. irritability or heightened awareness), tiredness, muscle pain, food cravings, or difficulties in thinking. Treating the attack during this period may reduce subsequent symptoms or even abolish them altogether. However, you should not use a triptan until the headache develops.

2.59 What is the migraine aura?

Only about one in 10 migraine sufferers get aura symptoms. These are usually short-lived, lasting up to 1 hour, and occur just before the migraine headache starts. Most aura symptoms are visual, including temporary blind spots, blurred vision, zigzag lines or flashing lights, but speech problems or tingling, loss of sensation and weakness in the arms and legs may also occur. Aura is caused by a spread of electrical activity in the brain. However, no damage occurs and there is no need to worry about it.

2.60 What are the symptoms of migraine?

The symptoms associated with an attack of migraine can vary considerably from patient to patient and from attack to attack, but generally evolve over time through a predictable pattern. After any warning signs and aura have passed, a headache generally begins as mild and diffuse but quickly becomes localised and moderate to severe in intensity. The headache usually throbs, is on one side of the head only and gets worse with physical activity. The headache is often accompanied by sensitivity to bright lights and loud noises, and sick feelings, which sometimes lead to vomiting. This headache phase normally lasts from 4 to 72 hours. After the headache, you might get hangover-like symptoms, which may linger for another day or two.

2.61 Does migraine impact on the lives of sufferers?

Migraine is an impactful condition. Attacks tend to prevent sufferers from conducting their normal employment, unpaid work and family and leisure activities. Migraine sufferers have poorer quality of life than the general population and, in severe cases, may experience problems in their employment and relationships with family and friends. However, with appropriate treatment, the vast majority of migraine sufferers can live normal lives and experience little disability.

2.62 Is migraine a genetic illness?

Migraine and tension-type headaches often run in families. The sufferer often finds that one or more of their relatives also has migraine, usually the mother, sister, aunt or grandmother, but sometimes also a male relative. It appears that genetic factors have a role in determining who gets migraine. Less commonly, migraine can occur after head or neck injury, psychological trauma, or infections. It therefore appears that many factors are involved in determining who gets migraine.

2.63 What causes migraine?

Migraine is a condition of the blood vessels and nerves in the brain. People with migraine have a nervous system that is susceptible to attacks. However, the attacks themselves tend to be triggered by something in the outside environment. When an attack is triggered, the so-called 'migraine generator' in the brain is activated. This leads to dilation of blood vessels and inflammation of nerves in the brain. In turn, this causes a nerve in the brain to fire (the trigeminal nerve), which causes the pain and other symptoms of the attack.

2.64 What are the symptoms of tension-type headache?

Tension-type headache is a nondescript headache with a dull and diffuse pain. The sufferer may also be sensitive to one of light or noise, but does not feel sick. Generally, this headache does not prevent the sufferer from conducting their normal activities.

2.65 What are the symptoms of chronic daily headache?

Chronic daily headache means frequent headache patterns occurring on more than 15 days per month with at least 4 hours of headache during each of these days. Normally, there is a low-grade near-daily headache with episodes of severe, more migraine-like headaches superimposed on top. Sufferers have often had migraine or tension-type headaches in the past, which evolve into chronic headache. Chronic daily headache may be caused by overuse of headache medications or may occur after a head injury.

2.66 Is migraine related to the menstrual period?

Girls and women who are menstruating frequently experience migraine near or at the time of their periods. A small proportion experience migraine only associated with their periods. Most doctors believe that the migraine attack occurs as the oestrogen levels rapidly fall at this time. Hormonal fluctuations are more correctly thought of as a trigger factor rather than as a direct cause of migraine.

2.67 I was recently diagnosed as having migraine. Is it safe for me to take the contraceptive pill?

You should talk to your doctor before starting the contraceptive pill, although in most cases there will be no problems. Women who have migraine without aura can safely take the contraceptive pill, unless their headaches worsen during treatment.

Most women having migraine with aura can also safely take the contraceptive pill but should be advised of the (very small) increased risk for stroke. It may be best for them to be given a pill with a low oestrogen dose. However, if the aura is prolonged and the woman has other risk factors, such as smoking, hypertension or hypercholesterolaemia, they should not take the contraceptive pill.

2.68 What are the migraine trigger factors?

Most migraine attacks occur spontaneously and there is little that can be done to prevent them. However, there is evidence that some factors may be involved in the triggering of migraine attacks. These factors include stress, hormonal changes in women, drinking red wine and head injury. Other factors that may lead to migraine include lifestyle and environmental changes, and certain foodstuffs, chemicals and drugs. Trying to reduce the incidence or effects of such factors may reduce the number of migraine attacks but is unlikely to abolish them altogether.

2.69 Can eating chocolate cause a migraine attack?

Many migraine sufferers believe that certain foodstuffs, and chocolate is chief among them, cause their migraine attacks. However, apart from the association with red wine, there is little evidence to support this link. Indeed, there is a more plausible explanation for this belief. Migraine sufferers often have cravings for certain foods or drinks during the prodrome phase of the migraine attack and consume chocolate and/or other foodstuffs. The chocolate may then be blamed for causing the headache when it appears a few hours later, when eating chocolate is actually more a consequence of the attack.

On the other hand, if you truly believe that eating chocolate can cause your migraine attacks, there is no harm whatsoever in cutting this, or any other, food from your diet.

Diagnosis of migraine and other headache disorders

3

MIGRAINE DIAGNOSIS

3.1 Are clinically valid guidelines for migraine diagnosis available to the physician?

Until relatively recently, uniform guidelines for the diagnosis of migraine were not available to the physician. Migraine was diagnosed in different ways in individual countries and even by individual physicians. The end result was that recognition and management of migraine were poor and worldwide estimation of migraine prevalence impossible. This problem was addressed in 1988 by the publication of definitive diagnostic guidelines by the International Headache Society (IHS). These guidelines have transformed research into migraine and the management of the condition by providing a standardised means of identifying migraine patients for physicians.

3.2 What are the International Headache Society guidelines for the diagnosis of migraine?

The IHS published comprehensive diagnostic criteria for migraine and other headache types. According to these criteria, migraine is a diagnosis of both inclusion and exclusion: inclusion because certain features must be present; and exclusion because secondary headaches must be eliminated as a prelude to diagnosis. Migraine is defined as shown in *Box 3.1*.

BOX 3.1 International Headache Society diagnostic criteria for migraine

- The occurrence of five or more lifetime headache attacks with similar features lasting from 4 to 72 hours each, patients being symptom-free between attacks (*these criteria help to exclude secondary headaches, which are less likely to recur without sequelae*).
- The presence of two or more of the following headache features:
- Moderate to severe pain
- Pain on one side of the head
- Throbbing or pulsating headaches
- Headaches exacerbated by routine activities (such as climbing stairs).
- The presence of one or more nonheadache associated symptoms:
- Aura symptoms (*see Q 3.3*)
- Nausea during the headache
- Photophobia and/or phonophobia during the headache.
- The exclusion of secondary headaches, by a search for 'headache alarms', by history taking or physical examination (*see Qs 3.6, 3.27–33*).

From the IHS diagnostic criteria, it is important to note that no single headache feature and no single nonheadache symptom are absolutely required for diagnosis. For example, a patient with severe bilateral headache associated with photophobia and phonophobia can be diagnosed with migraine, just like the more typical patient with unilateral, throbbing headache that is worsened by activity and accompanied with nausea. Migraine diagnosis using the IHS criteria is therefore somewhat of an art and requires a flexible approach rather than the simple 'ticking of boxes'.

3.3 How does the diagnosis of migraine with aura differ from that for migraine without aura?

For a migraine attack to be classified as migraine with aura, the IHS defines additional diagnostic criteria for the diagnosis of aura symptoms (*Box 3.2*).

BOX 3.2 International Headache Society diagnostic criteria for migraine aura

- One or more fully reversible aura symptoms (*see Q 2.15*).
- One or more aura symptoms develop gradually over more than 4 minutes, or two or more symptoms occur in succession.
- No single aura symptom lasts more than 60 minutes.
- The migraine headache occurs less than 60 minutes after the end of the aura symptoms.

In addition, secondary (sinister) headaches have to be excluded as the cause of the aura symptoms.

There are also several rare subtypes of migraine characterised by aura symptoms that differ from those described above. The diagnosis of these migraine subtypes is described later (*see Q 3.8*).

3.4 How does the diagnosis of migraine differ from that for 'migrainous' headache?

Migrainous headache attacks are those that do not quite meet the IHS criteria for any of the forms of migraine but which are classified as 'migrainous' in character. They are generally considered to be attacks of migraine. They are defined as headaches that meet all but one of the IHS criteria for migraine and do not fulfil the criteria for tension-type headache. For example, the patient may have a severe, bilateral headache associated with nausea and photophobia. Even though the patient only has one of the two headache characteristics prescribed by the IHS, their headache is certainly migrainous in character. This illustrates the fact that migraine diagnosis is not an exact science but requires the overall evaluation of a constellation of symptoms to arrive at an unequivocal diagnosis. The primary care physician should consider 'migrainous' headache to be a synonym for migraine.

3.5 Are these guidelines aimed at the specialist or primary care physician?

The IHS diagnostic guidelines were developed by a group of neurologists and headache specialists as a definitive means of diagnosing migraine and other headaches. They are now widely used by researchers for studies on migraine around the world and clinically in specialist neurology and headache clinics. Used appropriately, the IHS guidelines can be used to diagnose migraine definitively and differentiate it from other headache disorders.

However, full application of the IHS diagnostic guidelines is a lengthy process. Primary care physicians, who have severe restrictions on the time they can give to each patient, will often find them too cumbersome for routine use. Also, most headaches that primary care physicians encounter are due to the common disorders of tension type headache, migraine and chronic daily headache. Other headaches are rare and will be seen only occasionally, if ever. The primary care physician needs:

■ A means of identifying patients with rare or secondary (sinister) headache who are best referred to a specialist
■ A simple and rapid means of diagnosing migraine and other common headaches.

3.6 How can the primary care physician distinguish migraine from secondary (sinister) headaches needing referral to a specialist?

Although over 95% of the population experience headaches, a very small proportion of these headaches have sinister pathology. However, a critical aspect of diagnosing the symptoms of headache in the primary care setting is to separate primary headaches from headaches that are secondary to underlying disease. This is most efficiently accomplished by looking at the pattern of headaches a person presents with. In the medical setting a stable pattern (greater than 6-month history) of recurrent episodes of headaches that disrupt a person's function should be considered migraine until proven otherwise. The following data and observations support this statement:

■ Most significant sinister headaches are new in onset or differ from the established pattern of headache an individual experiences
■ Low impact headaches, unless chronic (not recurrent), do not reach a threshold where medical consultation is sought
■ People with migraine rarely have a stereotyped headache pattern but almost inevitably experience a variety of headache presentations from

migraine to migraine-like and tension type headache. All of these different presentations are reflections of the migraine process and respond in a similar fashion to migraine-specific medications.

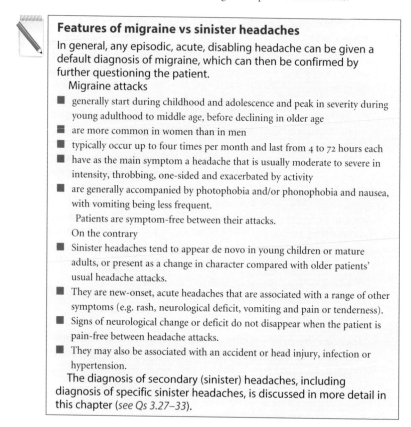

Features of migraine vs sinister headaches

In general, any episodic, acute, disabling headache can be given a default diagnosis of migraine, which can then be confirmed by further questioning the patient.

Migraine attacks

■ generally start during childhood and adolescence and peak in severity during young adulthood to middle age, before declining in older age

■ are more common in women than in men

■ typically occur up to four times per month and last from 4 to 72 hours each

■ have as the main symptom a headache that is usually moderate to severe in intensity, throbbing, one-sided and exacerbated by activity

■ are generally accompanied by photophobia and/or phonophobia and nausea, with vomiting being less frequent.

Patients are symptom-free between their attacks.

On the contrary

■ Sinister headaches tend to appear de novo in young children or mature adults, or present as a change in character compared with older patients' usual headache attacks.

■ They are new-onset, acute headaches that are associated with a range of other symptoms (e.g. rash, neurological deficit, vomiting and pain or tenderness).

■ Signs of neurological change or deficit do not disappear when the patient is pain-free between headache attacks.

■ They may also be associated with an accident or head injury, infection or hypertension.

The diagnosis of secondary (sinister) headaches, including diagnosis of specific sinister headaches, is discussed in more detail in this chapter (*see Qs 3.27–33*).

3.7 How can the primary care physician diagnose migraine rapidly and practically in their practice?

Making the initial diagnosis at the patient's first consultation is the first key step in the effective management of migraine. This can be accomplished simply and rapidly using the following scheme.

Migraine headaches are generally acute, painful and infrequent, and significantly affect the patient's quality of life and their ability to perform normal activities (*see Qs 2.25, 2.26*). In contrast, tension-type headache tends to not impact significantly on the patient's lifestyle (*see Q 1.14*) and chronic daily headache, by definition, is a chronic rather than an acute disorder (*see Q 1.17*).

A short series of four questions is useful to screen patients with headache at their first visit to the clinic (see *Fig. 3.1*).

1. What is the impact of the headache on the sufferer's daily life? (high impact = migraine or chronic daily headache; low impact = acute tension-type headache).
2. How many days of headache does the patient have every month? (≥ 15 days = chronic headache; ≤ 15 days = intermittent migraine).
3. For patients with chronic daily headache, on how many days per week does the patient take analgesic medications? (≥ 2 = analgesic-dependent headache; ≤ 2 = nonanalgesic-dependent headache).
4. For patients with migraine, does the patient experience reversible sensory symptoms associated with their attacks? (yes = migraine with aura; no = migraine without aura).

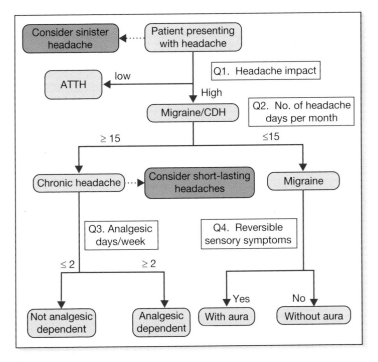

Fig. 3.1 Diagnostic scheme to screen for headache.

Two further brief investigations should be conducted in addition to these four questions:

A. Sinister headache should be considered, and eliminated, before asking the questions (*see Qs 3.6, 3.27–33*).

B. Once a pattern of chronic headaches is established (Question 2), the physician should investigate whether short-lasting headaches (e.g. cluster headache or short, sharp headaches) are the cause (*see Qs 3.17 and 3.15*).

BOX 3.3 A simple questionnaire to diagnose migraine designed for the primary care physician

Headache characteristics

■ Does the headache last between 4 hours and 3 days?
(a 'yes' answer is indicative of migraine)

■ Does the patient suffer from headache on more than 15 days each month?
(a 'yes' answer indicates chronic daily headache; a 'no' answer indicates an episodic headache disorder)

■ Does the patient feel well between attacks?
(a 'yes' answer is indicative of migraine)

■ Is the headache a throbbing, pulsating pain?
(a 'yes' answer is indicative of migraine)

■ Is the headache located on one side of the head at any stage?
(a 'yes' answer is indicative of migraine)

Nonheadache associated symptoms

■ Does the patient suffer from wavy lines, flashing lights or blind spots affecting their vision before or during the headache?
(a 'yes' answer is indicative of migraine with aura)

■ Does the patient feel sick or vomit during their headaches?
(a 'yes' answer is indicative of migraine)

■ Does the patient feel that they want to avoid light and/or noise during their headaches?
(a 'yes' answer is indicative of migraine)

Headache impact

■ Does the patient usually lie down when they have a headache?
(a 'yes' answer is indicative of migraine)

■ Is the patient prevented from, or have difficulties in, conducting their normal daily activities (employment, unpaid work and leisure activities) when they have a headache?
(a 'yes' answer is indicative of migraine)

Any high impact, intermittent, acute headache can therefore be given an initial default diagnosis of migraine and the IHS diagnostic criteria then be used to confirm this. Rather than using the IHS criteria as published, the physician can ask the series of questions shown in *Box 3.3*.

3.8 How can the rare migraine subtypes be diagnosed?

Some rarer migraine subtypes exist that are associated with abnormal aura symptoms:

MIGRAINE WITH PROLONGED AURA

This is a subtype of migraine with aura, where at least one aura symptom lasts for more than 60 minutes but less than 7 days. Most sufferers with this condition have normal duration auras for most attacks, with rare attacks of prolonged aura. Sufferers are rare who only experience prolonged auras. Acute onset prolonged aura may be indicative of transient ischaemic attacks or small strokes and should be investigated accordingly.

FAMILIAL HEMIPLEGIC MIGRAINE

Characteristic features of this subtype are auras that include hemiparesis, which may be prolonged, and having a first-degree relative who has the same condition. The condition probably has the same pathophysiology as migraine with aura and most sufferers experience mainly attacks of migraine with aura, with only a few attacks having associated hemiparesis.

BASILAR MIGRAINE

In this subtype, aura symptoms are present that clearly originate from the brainstem or the occipital lobes. Two or more of the following symptoms need to be present:

- Visual symptoms in both the temporal and nasal fields of both eyes
- Dysarthria
- Vertigo
- Tinnitus
- Decreased hearing
- Double vision
- Ataxia
- Bilateral paraesthesias
- Bilateral pareses
- Decreased level of consciousness.

The physician needs to evaluate these symptoms carefully as they may be indicative of anxiety and hyperventilation. Again, patients (who are mostly young adults) tend to have normal attacks of migraine with aura interspersed with attacks of basilar migraine.

MIGRAINE AURA WITHOUT THE HEADACHE

Attacks of migraine aura without subsequent development of headache are relatively common, especially as migraine sufferers get older. Sufferers who exclusively have such attacks are rare. Sufferers who develop these attacks for the first time at over 40 years of age should be investigated for possible transient ischaemic attacks.

RETINAL MIGRAINE

In this condition, repeated attacks of monocular scotoma or blindness lasting less than 1 hour are associated with headache. Patients have normal ophthalmological features outside these attacks. Ocular and structural vascular disorders need to be excluded for these patients.

MIGRAINOUS INFARCTION

In this condition, aura symptoms are not fully reversible over a 7-day period and/or are associated with ischaemic stroke confirmed by neuroimaging. Cerebral infarction may be linked to migraine in one of three ways:

- Cerebral infarction co-existing with migraine, but not related to it
- Cerebral infarction presenting with symptoms of migraine
- Cerebral infarction occurring during the course of a typical migraine attack.

Only the last of these definitions can be considered to be true migrainous infarction. An increased risk of stroke in migraine patients has not been demonstrated in epidemiological studies and stroke is a rare complication of migraine with aura, restricted to women aged under 45 years (see Q 2.10).

Other rare subtypes of migraine have abnormal symptoms associated with the headache phase of the attack:

OPHTHALMOPLEGIC MIGRAINE

In this condition, attacks of headache are associated with paresis of one or more cranial ocular nerves but without evidence of any intracranial lesion. The headache attacks may last for a week or more and their relationship to migraine is uncertain. However, this condition is extremely rare and may never be seen in normal primary care practice.

STATUS MIGRAINOSUS

In this condition, the headache phase of the migraine attacks lasts > 72 hours, despite treatment. Headache-free intervals of up to 4 hours may occur during this time. It is usually associated with prolonged drug use.

3.9 How can migraine aura symptoms be distinguished from sensory symptoms associated with an episode of epilepsy

Attacks of migraine without aura may be associated with epileptic seizures (*see Q 2.11*). Also, attacks of epilepsy with visual symptoms may be associated with headache that is very similar to migraine ('post-ictal headache'). Such attacks may be incorrectly diagnosed as being migraine with aura or as one of the rare migraine subtypes. However, the features of the visual symptoms of epilepsy are very different from those of migraine auras. If the patient has the following type of visual symptoms, a diagnosis of epilepsy can be confidently given:

- Symptoms usually last for seconds only
- Symptoms are mainly multiple, bright coloured, small circular spots, circles or balls
- Symptoms appear in a temporal hemifield, often moving contralaterally, or may be central in position and flashing
- Symptoms may multiply and increase in size during the seizure. Nonvisual occipital symptoms may develop, which rarely lead to extraoccipital symptoms and convulsions
- Patients with these symptoms have no family history of migraine.

These epilepsy symptoms are therefore different in colour, shape, size, location, movement and speed of development, duration and progress from those reported with migraine auras. This is important clinically, as treatment for epilepsy differs from that used for migraine with aura.

3.10 How can migraine in children be diagnosed?

Migraine presents in adolescents with similar symptoms to those reported by adults. The headache tends to be frontal, rather than one-sided, but nausea, photophobia and phonophobia are usually present. Typically, the patient goes to bed due to photophobia and phonophobia, goes to sleep and wakes up a few hours later with the attack resolved. In girls, initial migraine attacks may be associated with their menarche.

However, migraine may present with symptoms quite different from the usual in younger children. The characteristic symptoms of headache – nausea, photophobia and phonophobia – may be absent. Younger children may have brief, recurrent attacks of paroxysmal vertigo, causing them to lose their balance or be unable to walk, or a recurring pattern of cyclical vomiting. Older preadolescents may present with paroxysmal abdominal pain or recurrent episodes of limb pain. If patients present with these types of symptoms, together with a family history of migraine, then childhood migraine is the most likely diagnosis.

DIFFERENTIAL DIAGNOSIS OF MIGRAINE FROM OTHER PRIMARY HEADACHE DISORDERS

3.11 Is there a simple scheme that can be used to help with the diagnosis of different headache types?

A simple sequence of four questions can help the physician initiate diagnosis of their patients with headache, helping to differentially diagnose migraine from other episodic and chronic headache types. This scheme is described above (*see Q 3.7* and *Fig. 3.1*).

3.12 What is the 'spectrum' of headache?

Patients frequently have more than one type of headache and migraine and tension-type headache often coexist in the same patient. Patients' headaches exist in a continuum, ranging from pure migraine to pure tension-type headache, with predominantly migraine, half migraine and half tension-type headache and predominantly tension-type headache in between (*Fig. 3.2*). This diversity of presentation forms the 'spectrum' of headache that is encountered in clinical practice.

Interestingly, in patients who have migraine, all their headache attacks, including migraine, migrainous headache and tension-type headache, can

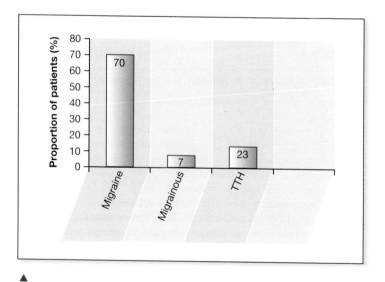

▲

Fig. 3.2 The spectrum of headache in migraine sufferers. Proportion of different headache types experienced by a population of 249 migraine sufferers.

be effectively treated with the triptan drugs. Triptans have a specific mechanism of action that targets migraine (*see* Q 4.30). They are relatively ineffective in the treatment of patients with pure tension-type headache. Therefore, these results indicate that all intermittent, acute headache presentations are manifestations of the migraine process in patients with migraine.

3.13 How can tension-type headache be diagnosed?

Tension-type headaches are recurrent episodes of headache that last between 30 minutes and 7 days. The headache is usually pressing or tightening in quality, of mild to moderate intensity, bilateral and does not worsen with physical activity. Sufferers do not experience vomiting but may report one (but not both) of photophobia or phonophobia.

Tension-type headache may be episodic (occurring on < 15 days per month) or chronic (occurring on ≥ 15 days per month). Nausea may be present during chronic, but not episodic, tension-type headache.

3.14 How can migraine be distinguished from tension-type headache?

Tension-type headache is often confused with migraine both by the patient and the physician. Key ways of distinguishing tension-type headache are as follows:

■ The headache is low-impact, patients being able to work and function fairly normally throughout the attacks. This is the key feature that distinguishes migraine from tension-type headache
■ The headache is typically bilateral, mild to moderate in intensity, and may persist for longer periods than migraine
■ Associated symptoms: one, but not both, of photophobia or phonophobia may be present, but these are usually mild in intensity
■ There is no associated vomiting, and nausea is only reported during chronic tension-type headache.

3.15 How can short, sharp headaches be diagnosed?

Features of the short, sharp headaches subtype include:

■ Patients are often young to middle-aged adults
■ The pain is piercing, very severe, short-lived, lasting from seconds to minutes (most commonly up to 30 seconds) and usually centred on one eye
■ Patients often feel slightly bruised after the pain has resolved
■ Patients can have multiple attacks during the day
■ The pain is frequently, but not always, triggered by eating ice cream or other cold foods.

Sometimes the headache lasts for over 3 minutes and diffusely affects one side of the head. This type of headache is termed *chronic paroxysmal hemicrania.*

3.16 How can migraine be distinguished from short, sharp headaches?

Patients and physicians may confuse short, sharp headaches with migraine due to their typical location on one side of the head. The key feature that distinguishes migraine from short, sharp headaches is their duration. Short, sharp headaches usually last from a few seconds to a few minutes only, while migraine attacks last from several hours to days. The headache is also different from migraine, with short, sharp headaches being piercing and neuralgic in quality.

Short, sharp headaches may also be confused with cluster headaches, due to their typical orbital location and the tendency for multiple daily attacks. Again, short, sharp headaches are shorter in duration than cluster headache attacks (15–180 seconds vs 15–180 minutes).

3.17 How can cluster headache be diagnosed?

Cluster headache is about five times more common in men than in women. The condition can be diagnosed if the following criteria are met:

- ■ The pain is excruciating (sometimes called 'suicide headache'), unilateral and often concentrated around one eye. One or more autonomic features are always associated with the headache; the eyes may be red and watering, and there is often a blocked nose. The pain is reported at the same site for all attacks.
- ■ Alcohol rapidly induces cluster headaches in most sufferers.
- ■ Each attack lasts from 15 minutes to 3 hours, with an average of 45 minutes (i.e. shorter duration than migraine). Attacks have an abrupt onset and cessation.
- ■ Attacks occur with a frequency ranging from once every other day to eight times daily. They often have a circadian rhythm, when they may be called 'alarm clock headache'.
- ■ Most patients (80–90%) have attacks that usually occur in clusters over the course of 2–3 months separated by attack-free intervals lasting from months to years (episodic cluster headache).
- ■ A minority of patients (10–20%) have symptoms for more than 1 year with pain-free periods of < 14 days (chronic cluster headache).

3.18 How can migraine be distinguished from cluster headache?

Migraine and cluster headache attacks have certain similarities but differ in several respects that make a differential diagnosis straightforward:

■ Cluster headache mostly affects men. Migraine mostly affects women.
■ During an attack period, cluster headaches are much more frequent than migraine attacks. The very frequent pattern of attacks is characteristic of cluster headache.
■ Cluster headaches are generally much shorter in duration than migraine attacks (15–180 minutes versus 4–72 hours).
■ The red and watering eyes and blocked nose often reported with cluster headache are not usually (but can be) reported with migraine.

3.19 How can chronic daily headache be diagnosed?

Although known under many names (*see Q 1.17*), chronic daily headache has the following characteristic features:

■ Very frequent headaches (> 15 days per month) lasting more than 4 hours
■ Headaches present for 6 months or longer
■ Headaches are resistant to treatment
■ A history of primary headache (migraine or tension-type headache) superimposed on a background of daily headaches
■ A possible history of head or neck injury
■ Likely chronic overuse of headache medications such as analgesics or ergots.

3.20 How can migraine be distinguished from chronic daily headache?

The continuum of different headaches that comprises chronic daily headache typically includes a background of migraine and/or tension-type headache attacks. Migraine therefore forms part of chronic daily headache for most sufferers. The key way to distinguish episodic migraine (or tension-type headache) from chronic daily headache is by recording the frequency of headaches. Chronic daily headaches (including chronic tension-type headache) are present on > 15 days per month, while migraine and episodic tension-type headaches are present on < 15 days per month – and usually considerably less frequent than this.

DIFFERENTIAL DIAGNOSIS OF MIGRAINE FROM SECONDARY HEADACHE DISORDERS

3.21 How can sinus headaches be diagnosed?

Key points of acute sinusitis allowing a correct diagnosis are:

■ Purulent discharge from the nose
■ Evidence of acute febrile illness

■ Headache in the sinus areas occurring simultaneously with the sinusitis
■ Dull, aching headache exacerbated by bending down
■ Diminished sense of smell.

A more severe form of sinusitis exists, called *pansinusitis*. This is a potentially serious condition that requires specialist intervention. It shares with acute sinusitis the features above, but in pansinusitis the pain is more generalized, rather than being confined to one of the paranasal sinuses.

3.22 How can sinus headaches be distinguished from migraine?

Acute sinusitis is a relatively uncommon cause of headache but is greatly over-diagnosed due to confusion with migraine and tension-type headache. A positive diagnosis of sinusitis is therefore required. Evidence of acute sinusitis, with a purulent discharge from the nose, and support with imaging or using a flexible scope, is required to confirm the diagnosis. In the absence of this evidence, migraine may be a more likely diagnosis. Also, in migraine the sense of smell is usually heightened, whereas in sinus headaches it is diminished.

3.23 How can trigeminal neuralgia be diagnosed?

Trigeminal neuralgia is the most common neurological syndrome in the elderly (approximately 155 in one million) and is three times more common in women than in men. Characteristic diagnostic features include:

■ Spasms of usually unilateral, intense, stabbing or burning pain along the trigeminal nerve lasting a few seconds to 2 minutes
■ Often provoked by activities such as washing, shaving, talking or brushing teeth
■ The patient is symptom-free between attacks.

3.24 How can trigeminal neuralgia be distinguished from migraine?

Trigeminal neuralgia shares certain features with migraine, e.g. it is more prevalent in women than in men, symptoms include severe, unilateral headache and the patient is symptom-free between attacks. However, two features distinguish it from migraine:

■ Trigeminal neuralgia typically affects the elderly, whilst migraine mostly affects young and middle-aged people
■ Attacks of trigeminal neuralgia are much shorter in duration than migraine attacks (< 2 minutes vs 4–72 hours)
■ The pain of the two types of headaches tends to be located at different sites: migraine pain is located in the temple and forehead; trigeminal neuralgia pain is located in the cheek and upper and lower jaws.

3.25 How can postherpetic neuralgia be diagnosed?

Postherpetic neuralgia is characterised by the presence of pain after an eruption of Herpes zoster. Care needs to be taken sometimes when the zoster rash is mild, hidden or absent or undetectable. Symptoms include a constant, deep pain with repetitive stabs or needle-prick sensations, starting during the acute rash. Light touch can trigger the symptoms and lead to itching. The condition has few similarities with migraine and there should be no difficulty in diagnosing between the two headache types.

3.26 How can temporomandibular joint dysfunction be diagnosed?

Temporomandibular joint dysfunction is characterised by:

- Noise in the joint on jaw movement
- Limited or jerky jaw movements
- Pain on jaw function
- Locking of jaw on opening
- Clenching and/or gnashing of teeth (especially teeth grinding whilst asleep)
- Tongue, lip or cheek biting or pressing.

This can lead to pain in the upper part of the head that is similar in character to migraine or tension-type headache. Patients prone to jaw clenching or teeth grinding while asleep may be prone to this syndrome. It is simple to distinguish patients with these jaw symptoms from other types of headache.

3.27 How can secondary (sinister) headaches be diagnosed?

Primary care physicians worry about misdiagnosing presenting headache symptoms as indicative of serious underlying pathology, although patients presenting with these conditions are rare. Patients, too, may be worried that their headache is caused by a brain tumour or other life-threatening disorder. However, the physician should realise that the majority of headache sufferers who seek advice have the common, high-impact headaches of migraine or chronic daily headache. Nevertheless, there are certain symptoms indicative of sinister headaches requiring referral that can be elicited straightforwardly by the primary care physician (*Box 3.4*). In general, sinister headaches, although constituting a vast minority of headaches reported, are generally new onset or different from the person's normal headaches.

Some examples of sinister headaches and their diagnostic pointers are shown in Box 3.4 below.

BOX 3.4 Diagnostic features suggestive of sinister headaches

Age
- Children: headache on wakening.
- Children: persistent headache.
- Older people: those having their first or worst headache at the age of > 50 years.

Features additional to the headache
- Pain or tenderness over the temporal artery, especially in patients > 50 years.
- Symptoms or signs additional to the headache, especially if they occur between the patient's headaches, e.g. progressive neurological symptoms.
- Headache following an accident or head injury.
- Headache with a rash, fever or stiff neck.
- Headaches (usually occipital) associated with uncontrolled hypertension.

Abrupt onset
- A sudden change in the patient's pattern of headaches.
- An acute onset of headache, especially when associated with vomiting.

3.28 How does headache related to meningitis present?

Headache related to meningitis infection is typically a new-onset acute headache in children that sometimes presents together with a rash (*Fig. 3.3*).

3.29 How does headache related to subarachnoid haemorrhage present?

Headache related to subarachnoid haemorrhage typically presents as a new-onset acute headache in people aged over 50 years with associated nausea and vomiting.

3.30 How does headache related to cranial arteritis present?

Cranial arteritis is typically seen in Caucasians aged > 60 years and Afro-Caribbeans aged > 50 years. It presents as a new headache with associated jaw pain, scalp and muscle tenderness and general malaise.

3.31 How does headache related to primary brain tumours present?

In primary brain tumours, headache is typically present together with symptoms or signs suggestive of neurological deficit between the headache attacks.

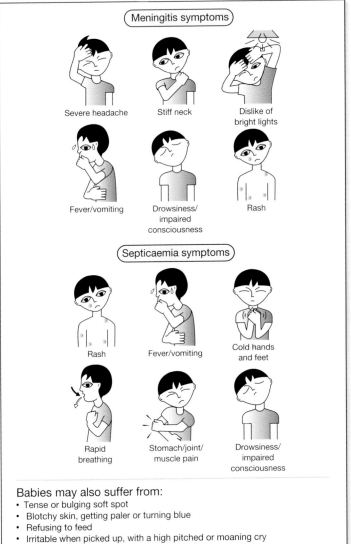

Babies may also suffer from:

- Tense or bulging soft spot
- Blotchy skin, getting paler or turning blue
- Refusing to feed
- Irritable when picked up, with a high pitched or moaning cry
- A stiff body with jerky movements, or else floppy and lifeless

Symptoms can appear in any order. Not everyone gets all these symptoms. Septicaemia can occur without meningitis.

Fig. 3.3 Key features suggestive of a diagnosis of meningitis. (© Meningitis Research Foundation, reproduced with kind permission)

3.32 How does headache related to cerebral metastases present?

Cerebral metastases may present in patients with a history of malignancy as headache together with neurological signs and/or deficit.

3.33 How does headache related to cerebral abscesses present?

Cerebral abscesses present as acute headache associated with neurological deficit, high or persistent fever and apparent infection of one or more systems.

PQ PATIENT QUESTIONS

3.34 Patient with migraine without aura

The patient is a schoolgirl aged 17 years. 'Doctor, I've been having headaches since I was 14. They occur every month just before my periods. The headache is usually throbbing, on the right side of my head and lasts for about 24 hours. I feel sick and bright lights, loud noises and cooking smells make it worse. What is wrong with me?'

Comment

This patient can be confidently diagnosed with migraine without aura. The symptoms of a throbbing, one-sided headache with associated nausea, photophobia and phonophobia alone are sufficient to make the diagnosis. The sociodemographic features of a female patient, headaches starting in the early teens and association of the headache with menstruation all help to confirm the diagnosis. However, the physician should realise that all diagnoses of migraine are not as straightforward as this one (*see Q 3.35*).

3.35 Patient with 'atypical' migraine symptoms

The patient is a 41-year-old man. 'Doctor, I get severe headaches about once every 3 months. They last for about 8 hours. The headache throbs and is on both sides of the head. I can't stand bright lights and have to lie down in a dark room till it goes away. What is wrong with me?'

Comment

Although the bilateral nature of the headache might be thought to indicate otherwise, this patient clearly has migraine. The presence of an acute, intermittent headache that interferes with the patient's normal daily activities (i.e. is disabling) suggests the default diagnosis of migraine. The presence of a severe headache with associated photophobia that forces the patient to lie down till he recovers is strongly suggestive of migraine.

3.36 Dealing with patient's fears of secondary (sinister) headaches

'I'm worried that the headaches I get might mean that I've got a brain tumour. How can I tell?'

Comment

Serious conditions such as brain tumours usually present with more symptoms than just a headache. If the patient has an established pattern of headaches, such as migraine or chronic daily headache, a new headache with similar symptoms is probably just another attack of their usual condition. However, if the patient develops new or unusual headache symptoms, they should be encouraged to discuss them with their physician.

3.37 Dealing with meningitis in a child

How can I tell if my child has meningitis?

Comment

Characteristic features of a child with meningitis include the following:

■ Severe headache
■ Stiff neck
■ Dislike of strong lights
■ Fever, with associated vomiting
■ Drowsiness and/or impaired consciousness
■ Rash – if a glass tumbler is pressed firmly against the rash, it will not
  fade and the rash can be seen through the glass (*Fig. 3.3*).

Not everyone gets all these symptoms and they may arise in any order. If
your child has these symptoms, call for medical help immediately.
For more information, contact the UK Meningitis Research Foundation at
www.meningitis.org
They also have a 24-hour helpline on 080 8800 3344.

3.38 Sinus headaches

'I have sinus problems and get really bad headaches about once a month. I
take painkillers but they do no good. What can I do?'

Comment

Many patients who think they have sinus headaches in fact have migraine. In
this case, the monthly frequency and severe intensity of the headaches
strongly suggest that migraine may be the cause of the patient's headaches.
The physician should institute a differential diagnosis procedure to ascertain
the true cause of these headaches.

3.39 Head splitting pains

'Doctor, I get really sharp pains in the side of my head, on one side. They
appear and disappear, but only last for a short time. Taking paracetamol is
no help at all. What have I got?'

Comment

Short, sharp headaches that are very intense but last for only a few seconds
are called 'ice cream' or 'ice pick' headaches. They are probably a type of
migraine. Patients should be reassured that these headaches are not sinister
and no specific therapy is required unless the patient insists. Due to their
short duration, acute therapy is unlikely to be successful anyway. If
necessary, preventative therapy may be called for and indomethacin is the
best medication to try first.

Migraine treatments

4

INTRODUCTION

4.1   How can migraine treatments be assessed and rated?

The rationale for this section is to provide objective evidence for the clinical profiles of drugs and nonpharmacological therapies used for the management of migraine in practice, both by physician interventions and by patients on their own or in concert with alternative practitioners. However, in the past it has been difficult to compare different therapies for headache and provide evidence-based guidelines for the choice of therapy to use. In general, there have been few well-controlled studies comparing different therapies and the type of headache in studies has often been poorly specified.

To achieve up to date, evidence-based recommendations for the treatments that have the best chance of success for the different patient populations who have migraine, evidence is analysed from the following sources, in order of importance:

■ Randomised, double-blind, placebo- or comparator drug-controlled clinical trials where the diagnosis of the headache was validated
■ Meta-analyses of controlled clinical trials
■ Less rigorously controlled clinical trials
■ Clinical practice guidelines in different countries
■ Consensus agreements from groups of physicians
■ From my own clinical experience.

I have drawn from the analyses conducted by the US Headache Consortium and published in the journal *Neurology* in 2000 (available on the American Academy of Neurology website at www.aan.com).

STRATEGIES FOR USING MIGRAINE THERAPIES

4.2   What are the strategies for treating migraine?

Medications for the treatment of migraine can be given in two ways:

■ Acute medication for the symptomatic treatment of individual attacks
■ Prophylactic medication to prevent the development of future attacks.

Medications can be prescribed or be available over the counter (OTC) without a prescription. The main classes of antimigraine drugs are available in most countries, although individual medications can differ in separate countries. Many antimigraine medications have their efficacy and safety profiles proven in controlled clinical trials. However, evidence for the utility of some of the older medications and the 'alternative' treatments tends to be much less robust.

'Alternative' therapies can also play a part, particularly for migraine prophylaxis. Lifestyle changes and behavioural therapies can be used as adjuncts to, e.g. reduce stress, alter the diet and change sleep patterns.

4.3 How should behavioural and lifestyle therapies be used?

Behavioural therapy should be part of managing all migraine patients. Wherever possible, this therapy should be used proactively and not instituted after everything else has failed. Behavioural therapy can be combined with drug therapy to achieve additional clinical effects.

4.4 How are acute management therapies chosen?

Acute medications are needed by all migraine sufferers for symptomatic treatment and, for the majority of patients who have infrequent attacks, are the only therapy required. It is therefore important that treatment is selected appropriate to the individual patient: their symptomatology, illness burden, impact on their daily lives and preferences all need to be taken into account.

Acute migraine therapies have not always been chosen systematically in the past and often a trial and error system has been used. One of three types of treatment strategy is typically used; step-care, staged care and stratified care (*Fig. 4.1*).

4.5 What is step-care?

In step-care, patients initiate treatment with one medication for a series of attacks. If this treatment fails, the physician can step the patient up to alternative, stronger medications for subsequent attacks. This stepping process continues until an effective medication is found or the patient gives up in disgust. In practice, patients are often given simple analgesics as first-line acute treatments. If these fail, they may be given a combination medication (e.g. an analgesic combined with an antiemetic). Specific migraine therapies, such as triptans and ergots, are often restricted to third- or fourth-line therapy when all other treatments have failed.

Step-care is ideal if the patient responds to the first-line simple analgesic, as this initial therapy is usually cheap and has few side effects. However, simple analgesics frequently do not work for migraine and most patients require a migraine-specific therapy. The result is that many patients will need repeated clinic visits and medication changes before an effective treatment programme is established. Patients and physicians may become discouraged during this process and the chances of the patients lapsing from care are high.

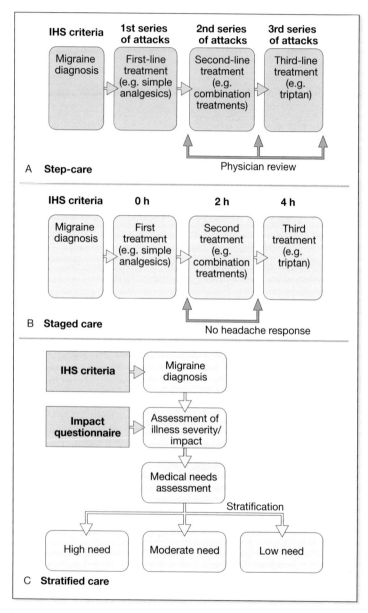

▲

Fig. 4.1 Strategies for the acute treatment of migraine: step-care, staged care and stratified care

4.6 What is staged care?

Staged care is a variant of step-care, where patients initiate treatment for each attack with a low-end medication. If this treatment fails, they can take stronger medications as rescue therapy. Again, patients commonly start with a simple analgesic but move up to combination and migraine-specific medications if this fails.

Staged care provides flexibility of treatment and gives the patient control over the medications they are taking. Rescue medication is always available to them if the initial treatment fails. However, the initial therapy is still unlikely to be effective for most migraine patients, who may experience significant suffering before they find effective treatment. In addition, the physician has no real control over what the patient is taking and may worry about the risk of overdosing.

4.7 What is stratified care?

In stratified care, the physician grades each patient as to the impact the migraine has on their lifestyle. This can be done using detailed history taking, or by using one of the new impact questionnaires, the Migraine Disability Assessment (MIDAS) questionnaire or the Headache Impact Test (HIT) (*see Qs 5.27–30*). The physician then prescribes therapy appropriate to the severity of the migraine. Patients suffering from little or no impact can be given simple analgesics or combination medications, while those with significant impact may be provided with migraine-specific therapies from the outset.

Stratified care increases the chances that the initial treatment will be effective, compared with step- or staged care. However, it allows little flexibility of use, and, if the initial treatment is ineffective, there may be no obvious fallback plan. Stratified care may also be expensive if patients are treating mild to moderate attacks with triptans, when a cheap combination analgesic may be effective.

4.8 What is the optimal strategy for using acute medications in primary care?

Migraine attacks are variable in frequency, duration and severity in the individual sufferer, as well as between different sufferers. Therefore, a single treatment is unlikely to be optimal for all attacks in each patient. Step-care is clearly not an option for this situation. To overcome this problem, a combination of stratified and staged care may work best. If the patient has access to a selection of medications, they can choose one appropriate to the severity of the current attack. Migraine sufferers can often predict the severity of an approaching attack based on their prior knowledge of premonitory symptoms.

In this scheme, the physician assesses the severity of the migraine and provides the patient with a range of medications, from simple analgesics to triptans. The patient then takes a triptan if the presenting attack is moderate to severe and a combination analgesic if it is mild to moderate. If either of these medications fails, the patient has rescue medication that they can take (usually a triptan). Such a scheme provides each patient with effective medications, and helps to ensure their use in a cost-effective way. The end result is individualised care that is patient focused and cost-effective.

4.9 How are prophylactic management therapies chosen?

Patients with frequent migraine attacks are usually also given a prophylactic medication. Although the definition of what constitutes 'frequent migraine' requiring prophylaxis varies in different countries, patients with three or more attacks per month in the USA or four or more attacks per month in the UK are usually given migraine prophylaxis. However, as all prophylactic agents have limited efficacy and have the risk of chronic side effects, an effective acute treatment is always required for the treatment of breakthrough attacks.

BEHAVIOURAL AND PHYSICAL THERAPIES FOR MIGRAINE

4.10 What are the behavioural and physical therapies for migraine?

Behavioural and physical therapies for migraine include the following:

BEHAVIOURAL THERAPIES

- Biofeedback and relaxation training, including hypnosis
- Cognitive-behavioural or stress management therapy
  - Development of coping skills
  - Cognitive restructuring, converting negative thoughts into positive messages
  - Assertiveness training
  - Goal identification
- Dietary therapy

PHYSICAL THERAPIES

- Manipulative procedures
- Massage
- Exercise: a routine of 20–40 minutes aerobic exercise per day
- Hyperbaric oxygen.

4.11 What are biofeedback and relaxation therapies?

Biofeedback is the process of bringing involuntary physiological functions under voluntary control. Biofeedback trains the nervous system to shut out excessive stimulation through calming music, visualisation and slow diaphragmatic breathing. With migraine, the aim is to reduce the level of central neuronal hyperexcitability, reducing the number of migraine attacks by ensuring, as far as possible, that the critical threshold for the development of the attack is not achieved. Standard biofeedback techniques used for migraine include thermal (hand warming) and electromyographic (EMG) biofeedback training.

Relaxation therapy is a simple technique that can be taught by any healthcare provider. It can be practised in groups without special equipment and is less costly and time consuming than any biofeedback technique. Relaxation techniques used for migraine include the control of muscle tension, mental relaxation and visual imagery to achieve treatment goals.

4.12 What is the evidence for the effectiveness of biofeedback and relaxation therapies for migraine?

Several studies support the use of biofeedback to prevent migraine attacks. However, relaxation therapy may be equally as effective as biofeedback.

Biofeedback has been shown to significantly improve migraine headaches, with a moderate to large effect. Thermal biofeedback and EMG biofeedback both improved the headache index (a combined measure of frequency and severity) by about 40% from pre- to post-treatment.

Relaxation training has also been shown to have a significant and moderately large effect on migraine frequency and severity. Results from 10 clinical studies showed a mean improvement of about 30–40% in headache frequency and headache index from pre- to post-treatment. Hypnotherapy has also been shown to reduce headache frequency.

Biofeedback has been frequently combined with relaxation therapy in studies. While this multitherapy was effective for migraine, there seemed to be no additive effects of combining the two therapies. Several studies have compared biofeedback plus relaxation therapy with prophylactic drugs for migraine. In general, the positive effects of these therapies were similar but additional efficacy was sometimes reported when the behavioural therapy was combined with the drugs.

4.13 What stress reduction strategies are used for migraine?

Migraine sufferers often feel responsible for their migraine and feel stress and guilt in being unable to control their attacks. They need to understand the mechanism of migraine and the fundamental role that an enhanced nervous sensitivity plays in it. Strategies used to reduce guilt and stress, and develop coping skills to confront migraine with a positive mental attitude include:

■ Cognitive restructuring: changing negative thoughts to positive messages
■ Assertiveness training: learning how to say 'no' to reduce guilt and stress
■ Identifying goals: establishing personal goals rather than relying on others to dictate behaviour.

4.14 What is the evidence for the effectiveness of stress reduction strategies for migraine?

Several studies have shown that stress reduction is an effective strategy to reduce the frequency and impact of migraine. There was a reduction in the number of attacks of approximately 50% and the effect was assessed as moderately large.

The combination of stress reduction and thermal biofeedback also reduced migraine frequency and severity. However, the effect seemed to be no larger than that reported for the two strategies given on their own.

4.15 What is the evidence for the effectiveness of dietary strategies for migraine?

Overall, the evidence that manipulating the diet can improve migraine frequency and symptomatology is poor.

Dietary strategies for migraine usually involve the removal of certain foods and drinks believed to trigger attacks. As we have seen (*see* Q 2.52), apart from red wine, there is no persuasive evidence that the exclusion of specific foodstuffs is of use in the treatment of migraine attacks. Indeed, one controlled study showed no relationship between eating chocolate and the precipitation of migraine attacks.

Increasing dietary riboflavin and magnesium has shown some efficacy in preventing migraine attacks (*see* Qs 4.118 *and* 4.119), which may be related to reduced levels of mitochondrial energy metabolism and brain magnesium in migraine, respectively.

One study has provided evidence that reducing the fat in the diet reduced migraine frequency, intensity and duration. However, this was an open study and further evidence is required from controlled clinical trials before the result can be confirmed.

4.16 What are the physical therapies used for migraine?

Several physical therapies have been used to treat migraine, including:

- Acupuncture, where the skin is pierced with fine needles to reduce pain and induce analgesia. The theory is that pain-killing endorphins are released
- Transcutaneous electrical nerve stimulation (TENS), where focused electric shocks are applied to areas of the body experiencing pain
- Occlusal adjustment, where dental procedures are used to improve the patient's bite, relieving muscle tension in the jaw that could possibly induce or worsen migraine pain
- Cervical manipulation, where short- or long-term high velocity thrusts are directed at joints of the cervical spine by a chiropractor, osteopath, physician or physiotherapist
- Hyperbaric oxygen, where the patient is placed in a hyperbaric chamber and administered oxygen to increase pressurisation of the blood gases
- Massage and exercise (a routine of 20–40 minutes aerobic exercise per day) as part of a stress-reduction strategy.

4.17 What is the evidence for the effectiveness of physical therapies used for migraine?

Acupuncture: the evidence for the efficacy of acupuncture as a migraine prophylactic agent is discussed in section *4.120*.

TENS: there is no good evidence that TENS has any effect on migraine. Two studies conducted to date showed that TENS was no better than subliminal TENS or sham TENS for the acute treatment of migraine.

Occlusal adjustment: only one study has investigated occlusal adjustment procedures for the prevention of migraine and no significant benefit was reported.

Cervical manipulation: several studies have shown that cervical manipulation can reduce the frequency, severity and associated disability of migraine attacks – although manipulation by a physician or physiotherapist was as effective as that by a chiropractor. There has been speculation that the cervical manipulation acts on physical conditions related to stress.

Hyperbaric oxygen: one small controlled study has investigated the effect of hyperbaric oxygen compared with oxygen given at atmospheric pressure (normobaric) for the acute treatment of migraine. The study showed that hyperbaric oxygen was significantly more effective than normobaric oxygen for the relief of migraine headache at 40 minutes after treatment. However, further large studies are necessary to confirm these findings. Also, even if there is a positive effect, use of hyperbaric oxygen would be severely limited due to the lack of general availability of suitable facilities.

4.18 Which of the behavioural and physical therapies can be recommended for migraine patients?

Biofeedback and physical therapies are a valuable adjunct to pharmacological therapies for migraine. Therapies that are recommended for the prophylaxis of migraine include:

■ Relaxation training
■ Biofeedback (thermal and EMG)
■ Combination of relaxation training and biofeedback
■ Stress reduction strategies.

There is no evidence that distinguishes between these different approaches to care and it is probably best if the patient chooses the therapies that appeal to them and are practicable. The great benefit of these therapies is that there are no associated side effects, meaning that they can be used with patients in whom prescribed drugs must be used with caution, e.g. children, pregnant women and older people with concurrent illnesses.

Patients may achieve additional benefits if the relaxation and biofeedback are combined with preventative drug therapy.

Cervical manipulation, massage and exercise may provide additional adjunctive therapy if used with other stress reduction strategies.

Dietary therapy, hypnosis, TENS, occlusal adjustment and hyperbaric oxygen cannot be recommended for the acute or prophylactic treatment of migraine at present, owing to the lack of available evidence.

ACUTE TREATMENTS FOR MIGRAINE

4.19 How do we evaluate the effectiveness of acute treatments for migraine?

Studies to evaluate acute treatments for migraine are now undertaken to unified and rigorous procedures to allow the evaluation of results into treatment guidelines and the comparison of different medications. In brief:

■ Studies are randomised, double-blind and placebo- or comparator-controlled
■ Patients are selected according to the IHS diagnostic criteria for migraine
■ The primary endpoint is headache relief, defined as a reduction from severe or moderate headache at baseline to mild or none at 2 hours after treatment
■ Other endpoints include improvement in headache to pain-free, improvement in nausea, vomiting and photophobia and phonophobia, improvement in the patient's functional abilities and the incidence of headache recurrence (where the headache is initially relieved at 2 hours, but subsequently deteriorates to severe or moderate over the 24-hour period after dosing).

4.20 What are the choices for acute treatments for migraine?

The commonly used acute treatments for migraine are listed below:

- Analgesics
  - Simple
  - Opiate
- Barbiturates
- Analgesic combinations
- Triptans
- Ergots
  - Ergotamine
  - Dihydroergotamine (DHE)
- Antiemetics.

ANALGESIC-CONTAINING PRODUCTS

4.21 Is paracetamol effective for migraine?

Migraine sufferers often try paracetamol as one of their first medications for migraine, due to its wide OTC availability. However, an evidence-based review of clinical studies conducted with paracetamol in migraine concluded that there was no objective evidence of its efficacy and it cannot therefore be recommended as monotherapy for migraine.

> Paracetamol is generally well tolerated, unless taken in large overdose, when it is dangerously hepatotoxic. It causes less gastric irritation than aspirin and the nonsteroidal anti-inflammatory drugs (NSAIDs).

4.22 Are aspirin and NSAIDs effective for migraine?

Aspirin and NSAIDs are usually among the first treatment that patients try for migraine, as they are freely available without a prescription. Clinical trials have shown that aspirin and certain NSAIDs (ibuprofen, naproxen sodium and tolfenamic acid) are effective for the treatment of mild to moderate attacks of migraine. About 40–50% of patients may report headache relief at 2 hours after treatment with these agents.

> Although these drugs are generally well tolerated, overuse can lead to analgesic-rebound headache and aspirin and NSAIDs can also cause gastrointestinal irritation, which can severely limit their use. The fact that these drugs can be used without any control from a

physician is a potential public health issue and undoubtedly contributes towards the development of chronic daily headache.

Aspirin and NSAIDs are inhibitors of COX-1 and this leads to the characteristic gastrointestinal side effects associated with their use. More recently, COX-2 inhibitors have been developed (e.g. rofecoxib) that are associated with much less gastrointestinal irritation than the COX-1 inhibitors. These drugs are used successfully for arthritis and are being investigated for migraine (see Q 8.8) but are not licensed for use in headache.

4.23   Are nonprescription combination analgesics effective for migraine?

Simple analgesics are often combined with other medications in an attempt to improve their efficacy for the acute treatment of migraine. Caffeine is added to attempt to improve the absorption of the analgesic and codeine is added to improve the analgesic power of the formulation. The combination of paracetamol 500 mg and codeine 8 mg is available in the UK OTC from pharmacists and is marketed to the general public as an effective treatment for migraine.

Clinical trial data have shown that the following combination medications are moderately effective and well tolerated for mild to moderate migraine:

- Aspirin plus paracetamol plus caffeine (available as Excedrin in the USA, but not the UK)
- Paracetamol plus codeine (available as Solpadeine in the UK).

In general, the nonprescription combination analgesics are well tolerated and have the same associated side effects as those of paracetamol and aspirin. However, codeine-containing preparations carry the risk of inducing chronic daily headache if used frequently and there are no controls to limit their use when bought OTC. The physician should investigate the usage of codeine-containing agents when patients present with a pattern of chronic headaches.

4.24   Are prescription analgesic-antiemetic combinations effective for migraine?

Simple analgesics are often combined with antiemetics in an attempt to improve their efficacy profiles for the acute treatment of migraine. Antiemetics such as domperidone and metoclopramide are added to prevent the gastric stasis often associated with migraine and to therefore improve the absorption of the analgesic. They may also reduce the nausea symptoms associated with migraine attacks.

Clinical trial data have shown that the following combination medications are moderately effective and well tolerated for mild to moderate migraine:

- Paracetamol plus domperidone
- Aspirin (as lysine acetylsalicylic acid) or paracetamol plus metoclopramide.

Approximately 40–50% of migraine patients report headache relief following treatment with these combination drugs. In a controlled clinical trial, the combination of paracetamol plus domperidone was shown to have similar efficacy to oral sumatriptan 50 mg in the treatment of moderate to severe migraine attacks.

Combinations of analgesics and antiemetics are all generally well tolerated. The combination of paracetamol and domperidone may cause raised serum prolactin, galactorrhoea, gynaecomastia, reduced libido, rash and allergic reactions. However, extrapyramidal symptoms (associated with antiemetics) are rare.

The combination of aspirin and metoclopramide may cause gastrointestinal upset and haemorrhage, drowsiness, endocrine disorders and extrapyramidal symptoms. The paracetamol and metoclopramide combination may cause extrapyramidal symptoms, raised serum prolactin, drowsiness and diarrhoea.

4.25 Are prescription combination isometheptene products effective for migraine?

The sympathomimetic isometheptene has been combined with paracetamol (plus sometimes dichlorphenazone) as an acute treatment for migraine. This combination has been shown to be significantly more effective than placebo for mild to moderate migraine in clinical trials. As with the NSAIDs and other combination medications, up to 50% of patients reported headache relief following the isometheptene drugs. One study showed that the combination of isometheptene, paracetamol and dichlorphenazone had similar efficacy to oral sumatriptan in the treatment of mild to moderate migraine attacks.

The isometheptene combination medications are well tolerated, with some drowsiness, dizziness, nausea and skin rash reported infrequently.

4.26 Are prescription opiate analgesics effective for migraine?

The combination of codeine (16–25 mg) with paracetamol has been shown to be effective for moderate to severe migraine in clinical trials and such combinations may be widely used. The OTC combination of paracetamol and codeine contains 16 mg of codeine in the recommended dose of two tablets, just within this therapeutic range.

Butorphanol nasal spray is used in some countries as a rescue medication for moderate to severe migraine when other treatments have failed. Clinical studies have demonstrated its efficacy in this role (*butorphanol is not licensed for migraine in the UK and Europe*).

Parenteral opiates (meperidine IM and methadone IM) are extremely effective pain killers and may be used as rescue medication for migraine in some emergency situations.

Side effects following codeine include dizziness, drowsiness, fatigue and nausea. Codeine is also a major cause of analgesic rebound headache and chronic daily headache. Its use, therefore, needs to be limited to avoid the development of dependency. This may be difficult to achieve if patients are taking OTC proprietary brands.

Side effects are also reported frequently with butorphanol and are similar to those described above for codeine. Again, frequent use can lead to analgesic rebound headache and chronic daily headache.

Parenteral opiates cause sedation, nausea and dizziness and carry the risk of abuse. Their use in migraine is restricted to the emergency room or other supervised settings where the sedation side effects will not put the patient at risk and where the risk of abuse can be addressed. There is concern in some countries about the numbers of patients who attend the emergency room to obtain opiate analgesics for their headaches. In fact, use of these rescue therapies should be discouraged due to the risk of development of chronic daily headache with analgesic dependence.

In conclusion, the risk of severe side effects means that the use of opiate analgesics for migraine should be restricted to supervised rescue therapy. While the occasional use of OTC codeine-containing products is unlikely to cause harm, patients who take them on more than two days per week on a regular basis are at risk of developing analgesic overuse and chronic daily headache. This is a potentially serious problem that is under-recognised by headache sufferers, physicians and healthcare policy makers.

4.27 Are barbiturate-containing products effective for migraine?

The combination of the hypnotic butalbital with aspirin, caffeine (and sometimes codeine) is available in some countries for the acute treatment of migraine. However, there is little clinical evidence for its effectiveness.

Barbiturate-containing products have significant side effects associated with their use. There are concerns over the side effects of drowsiness and sedation, with the risk of chronic overuse and associated rebound headaches and problems with withdrawal. Overdosing can also be dangerous. All these problems restrict the use of such products and they cannot be recommended for the acute treatment of migraine.

4.28 How can we recommend the use of analgesic-, isometheptene- and barbiturate-containing compounds for the acute treatment of migraine?

The following treatments have shown moderate efficacy in the acute treatment of migraine and can be recommended for treating mild to moderate attacks:

- Aspirin and other NSAIDs, in high doses
- Aspirin plus domperidone
- Aspirin (lysine acetylsalicylic acid) or paracetamol plus metoclopramide
- Isometheptene plus paracetamol-containing drugs.

Barbiturate-containing drugs should be avoided altogether and opiate-containing drugs restricted to supervised rescue therapy.

TRIPTANS

4.29 What are the triptans?

Triptans are migraine-specific medications. Triptans are agonists at the serotonin (5-hydroxytryptamine [5-HT]) 1B and 1D receptor subtypes. The first triptan was sumatriptan, developed during the late 1980s and marketed since the early 1990s in most countries around the world. Sumatriptan was developed following the observation that levels of serotonin were reduced during migraine attacks and that treatment with it could ameliorate attacks. Unfortunately, serotonin was associated with too many side effects to be practicable for use in clinical practice. Sumatriptan was developed to mimic the antimigraine effect of serotonin but without significant side effects.

4.30 What is the mode of action of the triptans?

Triptans act as agonists at the $5\text{-HT}_{1B/1D}$ receptor and have a dual mechanism of action against migraine. They have a selective vasoconstrictor action on dilated cranial blood vessels, returning them to their normal size, and also act on trigeminal nerve terminals, reducing neuronal firing and the release of inflammatory factors. Both of these mechanisms result in a reduced stimulation of the trigeminal nerve and amelioration of all migraine symptoms: headache, photophobia and phonophobia, and nausea and vomiting (*see* Q 2.42).

All triptans act on blood vessels and nerve endings in the brain. However, they are lipophilic to different extents. Some can penetrate the blood–brain barrier and also act significantly on central 5-HT_1 receptors. The clinical significance of this effect is uncertain, as the lipophilic triptans are not noticeably more effective than the nonlipophilic drugs.

Triptans selectively constrict blood vessels in the brain, which contain the 5-HT 1B and 1D receptors. Peripheral blood vessels, e.g. those in the heart, have a very low concentration of these receptors and the vasoconstrictor effect of triptans at these sites is low and, except in very rare cases, clinically insignificant.

4.31 What triptan drugs and formulations are available to the physician?

Seven triptans are now available to the physician or have been approved by regulatory agencies in at least some countries:

1. Sumatriptan (Imigran, Imitrex in the USA and some other countries): available in oral (conventional tablet), nasal spray, subcutaneous and, in a few countries, suppository formulations
2. Naratriptan (Naramig, Amerge in the USA): available in an oral (conventional tablet) formulation
3. Zolmitriptan (Zomig): available in oral (conventional and orally-disintegrating tablet [ODT]) formulations and submitted for regulatory approval as a nasal spray formulation
4. Rizatriptan (Maxalt): available in oral (conventional and ODT) formulations
5. Almotriptan (Almogran, Axert in the USA): available in an oral (conventional tablet) formulation
6. Eletriptan (Relpax): available as an oral (conventional tablet) formulation
7. Frovatriptan (Elan): recently approved by the US FDA in an oral (conventional tablet) formulation.

More triptans are still in clinical development and are likely to be introduced over the next few years, e.g. donitriptan.

4.32 What are the features of the efficacy profile shared by all the triptans?

All of the available triptans share many clinical features:

■ They are effective acute treatments for moderate to severe migraine, relieving the headache and nonheadache migraine symptoms (nausea, vomiting, photophobia and phonophobia). Owing to this feature, no added antiemetic is required.

■ Triptans are equally effective for the treatment of migraine with aura and migraine without aura.

■ For oral triptans, efficacy starts within 1 hour of dosing and increases up to 2–4 hours. Typically, 60% or more of patients report headache relief by 2 hours after treatment. Nasal spray and subcutaneous formulations produce a greater response and have a more rapid onset of action. Studies suggest that administration of triptans while the pain is mild increases their efficacy.

■ Triptans are effective in long-term clinical use, with about 80% of attacks being relieved at 2 hours after treatment. Efficacy in clinical practice is typically greater than that reported in controlled clinical trials.

■ Headache recurrence is reported by about 30% of patients in the 24 hours following triptan dosing, necessitating a second dose. Studies demonstrate lower recurrence when migraine pain is resolved rather than just relieved.

■ Triptans improve the QOL of migraine patients and their use is cost-effective. Cost savings are frequently reported for triptans compared with other treatments.

Triptans are generally well tolerated, with adverse events being short-lived, mild to moderate in intensity and characteristic of the class of drugs, including:

■ Unpleasant but short-lived feelings of pain, heaviness or tightness in any part of the body, including areas such as the chest and neck, which can alarm the patient

■ Nausea

■ Drowsiness and fatigue

■ Dizziness.

As with the ergots (*see Q 4.80*), there is the potential for vasoconstriction of coronary arteries and triptans are contraindicated for patients with risk factors for cardiovascular disease. If angina-like symptoms (transient chest pain or throat symptoms) occur, the triptan should be withdrawn and the cause investigated. However, triptans are shorter-acting than ergots, the cardiac vasoconstriction is much less and the risk of cardiovascular adverse events is low. For example, sumatriptan has been shown to be well tolerated in the treatment of over 300,000 migraine attacks in clinical trials and over 200 million attacks in clinical practice. Significant cardiovascular and cerebrovascular events were only rarely reported.

Owing to the potential for interactions between triptans and other drugs, triptans are contraindicated for use in patients taking certain other drugs. Specific contraindications are dealt with below for each triptan in turn but most triptans are contraindicated for use with monoamine oxidase inhibitors (MAOIs), other triptans and ergotamine and its derivatives.

4.33 How cost-effective are the triptans?

Triptans are relatively expensive drugs, particularly when compared with more traditional therapies – which are mostly off-patent and therefore cheap. Numerous economic studies have consequently been conducted to establish the cost-effectiveness of the triptans against previously used therapies, most of these being conducted with sumatriptan.

Controlled clinical studies generally show that the introduction of a triptan considerably increases the direct costs of medical therapy for migraine. Although the number of consultations for migraine declines, this is more than offset by the increased costs of procuring the triptan. However, the increased direct costs are more than balanced by savings in indirect costs due to reduced absence from work and productivity losses. Triptans are therefore cost-effective to use. The fact that triptans are significantly more effective than conventional therapies in reducing patients' migraine symptoms, disability and improving quality of life reinforces the significance of these results.

SUMATRIPTAN

4.34 What are the pharmacological features of sumatriptan?

Sumatriptan was the first of the triptans to be developed and has the largest portfolio of clinical data of all the triptans. It is fairly rapidly absorbed and excreted (Tmax and $T\frac{1}{2}$ both within 2–3 hours) but has low bioavailability (15%) and minimal central nervous system penetration (*Table 4.1*). It is available as 25 mg (USA only), 50 mg and 100 mg (not in USA) conventional tablets, 5 mg and 10 mg (USA only) and 20 mg nasal sprays, 6 mg subcutaneous injections and 12.5 mg and 25 mg suppositories (not in the UK and the USA). The clinical profile has been elucidated for all four formulations.

TABLE 4.1 Pharmacological profiles of the oral triptans. Of the triptans below, sumatriptan penetrates the central nervous system (CNS) to the least extent

Triptan	Absorption Tmax (h)	Plasma half-life $T^{1}/_2$ (h)	Bioavailability (%)
Sumatriptan	2.5	2.5	15
Naratriptan	2–4	5.6–6.3	63–74
Zolmitriptan	2	2.5–3	40–48
Rizatriptan	1–1.5	2–3	45
Almotriptan	1.4–3.8	3.2–3.7	70
Eletriptan	1–2	3.6–5.5	50
Frovatriptan	2–4	25	24–30

4.35 What special precautionary measures must be taken with sumatriptan?

Sumatriptan is *contraindicated* for use in patients with ischaemic heart disease, previous myocardial infarction, cerebrovascular accident, Prinzmetal's angina, uncontrolled hypertension, coronary vasospasm and severe hepatic impairment.

Special *precautions* must be taken when sumatriptan is given to patients with cardiac diseases and those having risk factors for coronary artery disease, hepatic or renal impairment, controlled hypertension, sensitivity to sulphonamides, women who are pregnant or lactating and people driving or operating machinery.

Sumatriptan may *interact* with MAOIs, 5-HT re-uptake inhibitors and ergotamine.

4.36 How effective is oral sumatriptan?

Controlled clinical trials have shown that all oral doses of sumatriptan are significantly superior to placebo for the acute treatment of migraine. The proportion of patients who reported headache relief (severe or moderate headache improving to mild or none after 2 hours) were 56–62% for the 100 mg, 50–61% for the 50 mg and 52% for the 25 mg doses (*Table 4.2*) In a comparison study of the three doses, the 50 mg and 100 mg were equivalent in efficacy and significantly superior to the 25 mg.

Recent studies have demonstrated that migraine sufferers with significant migraine-related disability have multiple clinical presentations of their migraine attacks (migraine, tension-type headache and migrainous headache [*see Q 3.12*]) and that the entire spectrum of this headache activity is effectively treated by oral sumatriptan 50 mg. In addition, intervention in a migraine attack during the mild headache phase significantly improves

TABLE 4.2 Summary of the clinical profiles of the different triptan drugs from randomised, placebo-controlled clinical trials

Triptan	Dose and route of administration	ARR (%)	PRR (%)	TG (%)	NNT
Sumatriptan	6 mg subcutaneous	81–82	31–39	43–50	2.0–2.3
Sumatriptan	100 mg oral	56–62	17–26	30–40	2.5–3.3
Sumatriptan	50 mg oral	50–61	17–27	24–37	2.7–4.2
Sumatriptan	25 mg oral	52	17–27	25–35	2.9–4.0
Sumatriptan	20 mg nasal spray	55–64	25–36	24–39	2.6–4.2
Sumatriptan	12.5 mg suppository	43–69	21–48	0–48	2.1–∞
Sumatriptan	25 mg suppository	64–74	21–48	16–53	1.9–6.3
Naratriptan	2.5 mg oral	43–50	18–27	16–28	3.6–6.3
Zolmitriptan	2.5 mg oral	62–65	34–36	25–31	3.2–3.8
Zolmitriptan	2.5 mg ODT	63	22	41	2.4
Zolmitriptan	5 mg nasal spray	70	30	40	2.5
Rizatriptan	10 mg oral	67–77	35–40	27–40	2.5–3.7
Rizatriptan	10 mg ODT	74	28	46	2.2
Almotriptan	12.5 mg oral	57–65		14–33	3.0–7.1
Eletriptan	40 mg oral	62–65	19–24	41–43	2.3–2.4
Eletriptan	80 mg oral	65–77	19–24	46–53	1.9–2.2
Frovatriptan	2.5 mg oral	36–46		13–19	5.3–7.7

ARR = triptan response rate: PRR = placebo response rate (percentage of patients who improved from severe or moderate headache pain to mild or none 2 hours after treatment.

TG = therapeutic gain (ARR minus PRR)

NNT = number needed to treat (the number of patients it is necessary to treat to achieve one patient with a successful response, adjusted for placebo)

efficacy and reduces headache recurrence. Finally, these studies suggest that disabling episodic tension-type headache is uncommon in clinical practice and that migraine attacks, while they may begin with mild symptoms, very frequently evolve into moderate to severe headache.

Oral sumatriptan is effective in treating menstrual migraine attacks in women but is relatively ineffective in treating migraine in children.

Oral sumatriptan is generally well tolerated in clinical studies and clinical practice. Reported adverse events include pain, sensations of heaviness and pressure in any part of the body, fatigue, dizziness, drowsiness, weakness and increases in blood pressure. Reports of seizures, hypotension, bradycardia, serious coronary events and hypersensitivity reactions are rare.

Due to its low lipophilicity and consequent poor ability to penetrate centrally, sumatriptan has a low potential to cause CNS adverse events, such as dizziness and somnolence.

4.37 How effective is nasal spray sumatriptan?

Controlled clinical trials have shown that 5, 10 and 20 mg doses of sumatriptan nasal spray are significantly superior to placebo for the acute treatment of migraine. The 20 mg dose is optimal, with 55–64% of patients reporting headache relief after 2 hours (*Table 4.2*). The overall response to sumatriptan nasal spray is similar to that for the oral formulation but there is a faster onset of action (within 15 minutes of treatment). Nasal spray sumatriptan was shown to be an effective treatment for migraine attacks in adolescents and younger children (aged 5–12 years), who tend to be resistant to triptan therapy.

> Nasal spray sumatriptan is generally well tolerated in clinical studies and in clinical practice and adverse events are similar to those reported for oral sumatriptan (*see Q 4.36*). However, the most frequently reported adverse event following sumatriptan nasal spray is a taste disturbance caused by the bitterness of the formulation. A new delivery device for nasal spray sumatriptan is in development which may result in improved tolerability of this formulation.

4.38 How effective is subcutaneous sumatriptan?

Controlled clinical trials have shown that subcutaneous sumatriptan 6 mg is significantly superior to placebo for the acute treatment of migraine, with 81–82% of patients reporting headache relief after 2 hours (*Table 4.2*). There is a very fast onset of action, within 10 minutes of treatment. Subcutaneous sumatriptan is clearly the most effective of all the triptan formulations.

Subcutaneous sumatriptan effectively treats menstrual migraine attacks, early-morning migraine, and attacks in migraine sufferers with drug-withdrawal headache. It is also a very effective treatment for cluster headache (*see Q 4.126*).

> Subcutaneous sumatriptan is generally well tolerated with a similar pattern of adverse events as the oral formulation (*see Q 4.36*). However, it is associated with more adverse events than for the oral and nasal spray and suppository formulations, especially flushing, dizziness/vertigo and paraesthesia/tingling. In addition, pain and irritation at the injection site are frequently reported. A needle-less injector is currently in development and should minimise these latter effects once it is introduced.

4.39 How effective is the suppository formulation of sumatriptan?

Sumatriptan suppository is not widely available but is marketed in Germany, Sweden, Switzerland and Greece. Controlled clinical trials have shown that sumatriptan suppository 12.5 mg and 25 mg are significantly superior to placebo for the acute treatment of migraine, with 43–69% of patients reporting headache relief after 2 hours with the 12.5 mg dose and 64–74% with the 25 mg dose (*Table 4.2*). There is an onset of action within 30 minutes of treatment.

> Sumatriptan suppository is very well tolerated with the overall profile of adverse events in clinical studies being similar to that reported for placebo. The pattern of adverse events reported in clinical practice is generally the same as that reported for oral sumatriptan (*see Q 4.36*). Anorectal events, such as burning, itching or irritation are rare, being reported by < 1% of patients in clinical studies.

4.40 How does sumatriptan compare with other acute migraine therapies?

Numerous clinical studies have shown that oral and subcutaneous formulations of sumatriptan are significantly superior to nontriptan medications traditionally used for the acute treatment of migraine. A controlled comparator clinical study showed that oral sumatriptan 100 mg was significantly superior to oral ergotamine plus caffeine (Cafergot). However, comparisons with analgesic combination medications were more equivocal. One study with aspirin plus metoclopramide showed that sumatriptan 100 mg was superior but a second study with aspirin plus metoclopramide and a study with an NSAID (rapid-release tolfenamic acid) showed no significant differences between the treatments.

Studies have shown that subcutaneous sumatriptan 6 mg is superior to oral sumatriptan and to subcutaneous and nasal spray DHE. Nasal spray sumatriptan 20 mg was also shown to be significantly more effective than nasal spray DHE. However, sumatriptan suppository was less effective than a suppository formulation of ergotamine (*see Q 4.83*).

Sumatriptan has long been the gold standard for acute migraine therapy, as it was the only available triptan for several years. The newer triptans have all conducted comparator studies with sumatriptan and these are discussed below (*see Qs 4.45, 4.52, 4.58, 4.63, 4.68 and 4.73*).

4.41 How can sumatriptan be recommended as an acute treatment for migraine?

Sumatriptan has now been used for over a decade in clinical practice, where the favourable clinical profile established in clinical trials has been corroborated and reinforced. The portfolio of formulations and doses provides the physician with flexible therapy that can be tailored to the patient's requirements and preferences. All formulations of sumatriptan can therefore be recommended as first-line acute treatments for migraine.

NARATRIPTAN

4.42 What are the pharmacological features of naratriptan?

Naratriptan has a longer half-life (5.6–6.3 hours) and much higher oral bioavailability (63–74%) than most other triptans (*Table 4.1*), which may promote a more sustained effect. Naratriptan is available as a 2.5 mg conventional tablet.

4.43 What special precautionary measures must be taken with naratriptan?

Naratriptan is *contraindicated* for use in patients with ischaemic heart disease, previous myocardial infarction, a history of cerebrovascular accident or transient ischaemic attacks, Prinzmetal's angina, peripheral vascular disease, uncontrolled hypertension, coronary vasospasm and severe renal and hepatic impairment.

Special *precautions* must be taken when naratriptan is given to patients at risk of coronary artery or cardiac diseases, patients with mild to moderate hepatic or renal impairment, sensitivity to sulphonamides and women who are pregnant or lactating.

Naratriptan may *interact* with other 5-HT$_1$ agonists, methysergide and ergot derivatives.

4.44 How effective is oral naratriptan?

Naratriptan was shown to be significantly superior to placebo as an acute treatment for migraine. At first glance, naratriptan appears to be one of the least effective of the triptans, with 43–50% of patients reporting headache relief 2 hours after treatment. However, its full efficacy is not reported until 4 hours, when 60–68% of patients report headache relief (*Table 4.2*). The efficacy of naratriptan is maintained over a 24-hour period following treatment and it has one of the lowest reported recurrence rates of any triptan (19–28%).

Owing to its long action, naratriptan has been investigated as a preventative or prophylactic drug for several headache subtypes. Studies have shown that it may be effective for:

- The prophylaxis of transformed migraine (a type of chronic daily headache) when given at a dose of 2.5 mg/day

- The short-term prophylaxis of menstrually associated migraine when given at a dose of 1 mg twice daily during the perimenstrual period
- The prevention of migraine when given at a dose of 2.5 mg during the prodrome phase of the attack
- The prophylactic treatment of cluster headache.

While naratriptan shows promise in all these areas, further studies are required to confirm these clinical effects before it can be generally recommended.

> Naratriptan is very well tolerated with the profile of adverse events being similar to that reported for placebo. Adverse events that have been reported include malaise, fatigue, dizziness, nausea, pain or sensations of warmth, heaviness or pressure in any part of the body (including the throat or chest), bradycardia and visual disturbances.

4.45 How does naratriptan compare with other migraine therapies?

Naratriptan is clearly superior to nontriptan acute medications for migraine. Patients who had been taking simple analgesics, combination products and narcotics reported greater pain relief and an increased ability to function when they were switched to naratriptan.

Naratriptan may be associated with less headache recurrence than some other triptans. The incidence of headache recurrence was compared after treatment with naratriptan 2.5 mg and sumatriptan 100 mg in a population of patients with a history of frequent headache recurrence. Fewer patients reported recurrence after naratriptan than after sumatriptan (recurrence after one attack: 45% vs 57%, not significant; recurrence after two attacks: 41% vs 57%, $P < 0.01$). In addition, the incidence of adverse events was lower with naratriptan than with sumatriptan (22% vs 33%).

The sustained efficacy of naratriptan may be similar to that of other triptans. The 4-hour efficacy of naratriptan 2.5 mg was shown to be less than that of sumatriptan 100 mg (headache relief: 63% vs 80%, $P < 0.05$). However, efficacy at 24 hours was similar for the two treatments and naratriptan was associated with fewer episodes of headache recurrence and adverse events.

Naratriptan 2.5 mg was shown to be an effective treatment for patients who were nonresponders to sumatriptan 50 mg.

4.46 How can naratriptan be recommended as an acute treatment for migraine?

Naratriptan is an effective and well tolerated acute treatment for migraine but has a slower onset of action and a lower 2- and 4-hour response rate than most other triptans. It may be recommended as a first-line therapy for patients who do not require a fast-acting therapy or who are afraid of the usual triptan adverse events. It can also be recommended as a very useful second-line therapy for patients who have reported regular headache recurrence and/or unpleasant side effects, or who are nonresponders to previous triptan therapy.

ZOLMITRIPTAN

4.47 What are the pharmacological features of zolmitriptan?

Zolmitriptan is absorbed rapidly (Tmax = 2 hours) and has a high bioavailability (40–48%) (*Table 4.1*). It is more lipophilic than sumatriptan and penetrates the central nervous system to a significant extent. It is available as 2.5 mg conventional and orally-disintegrating tablets (ODT). Patients take a single 2.5 mg tablet to treat their attacks but can increase the dose to 5 mg for subsequent attacks if this dose is not effective. Zolmitriptan has also been approved as a 5 mg nasal spray in several markets.

4.48 What special precautionary measures must be taken with zolmitriptan?

Zolmitriptan is *contraindicated* for use in patients with ischaemic heart disease, coronary vasospasm, Prinzmetal's angina, Wolff-Parkinson-White syndrome, arrhythmias associated with other accessory pathways and uncontrolled hypertension.

Special *precautions* must be taken when zolmitriptan is given to patients with risk factors for ischaemic heart disease or with hepatic impairment, those who are hypersensitive to zolmitriptan and women who are pregnant or lactating.

Zolmitriptan may *interact* with other 5-HT_1 agonists, ergotamine, moclobemide, MAOIs, cimetidine, fluvoxamine and quinolones.

4.49 How effective is oral zolmitriptan?

Oral zolmitriptan was shown to be significantly superior to placebo for the acute treatment of migraine with an onset of action within 45 minutes of administration. For the conventional tablet, the efficacy of the two doses was similar in clinical trials, with 62–65% of patients receiving the 2.5 mg dose and 59–67% of those receiving the 5 mg dose reporting headache relief 2 hours after treatment (*Table 4.2*). The 2.5 mg dose was also effective in treating menstrually-associated migraine attacks and attacks in adolescent migraine sufferers.

Oral zolmitriptan is generally well tolerated, although more adverse events are reported following the 5 mg than the 2.5 mg dose. Adverse events reported include nausea, dizziness, warm sensations, dry mouth, asthenia, somnolence, heaviness or pressure in the throat, neck, limbs and chest, myalgia, muscle weakness and paraesthesia.

4.50 How effective is zolmitriptan orally-dispersible tablet?

The 2.5 mg ODT formulation of zolmitriptan is a nonfriable orange-flavoured tablet. This formulation was shown to have a similar clinical profile to the conventional tablet. In a placebo-controlled study, 63% of patients reported headache relief after 2 hours, with an onset of action within 1 hour (*Table 4.2*). The majority of patients (70%) preferred the ODT to the conventional tablet.

 The ODT formulation of zolmitriptan was well tolerated with an adverse event profile similar to that of the conventional tablet (*see Q 4.49*).

4.51 How effective is nasal spray zolmitriptan?

Zolmitriptan nasal spray was apparently more effective than the oral formulations when administered at a dose of 5 mg. In a placebo-controlled, multiple-attack study, 70% of patients reported headache relief after 2 hours with an onset of action within 15 minutes (*Table 4.2*). Consistency of response was also good with 74% of patients responding in two or three of the three attacks treated.

The nasal spray formulation of zolmitriptan was well tolerated in long-term use. However, full tolerability and safety data for nasal spray zolmitriptan have yet to be reported.

4.52 How does zolmitriptan compare with other migraine therapies?

Oral zolmitriptan appears to have a very similar clinical profile to oral sumatriptan. An international study showed that zolmitriptan 2.5 mg and 5 mg doses had similar efficacy profiles to sumatriptan 50 mg. At 2 hours, headache relief was reported by 63%, 66% and 67% of patients receiving zolmitriptan 2.5 mg and 5 mg, and sumatriptan 50 mg, respectively. Headache recurrence and adverse event rates were also similar in the three groups.

In a crossover, patient preference study with zolmitriptan 2.5 mg and sumatriptan 50 mg, 44%, 27% and 27% of the patients preferred zolmitriptan, sumatriptan and had no preference, respectively. A faster onset of action was the most important reason for preference given for both triptans.

4.53 How can zolmitriptan be recommended as an acute treatment for migraine?

Zolmitriptan is an effective and well tolerated acute treatment for migraine. The conventional tablet and ODT oral formulations have very similar clinical profiles to that of oral sumatriptan and can be recommended as first-line acute treatments for migraine. The ODT formulation may be particularly suitable for patients who have unpredictable attacks and need to take their medication at any time or place.

Nasal spray zolmitriptan seems to be slightly more effective and have a faster onset of action than the oral zolmitriptan formulations. Although its full clinical profile is not yet established, it may be particularly suitable for patients who have unpredictable severe attacks that require rapid treatment.

RIZATRIPTAN

4.54 What are the pharmacological features of rizatriptan?

Rizatriptan is a potent and selective $5-HT_{1B/1D}$ receptor agonist that, like zolmitriptan, can act centrally as well as peripherally on receptors. It has a relatively high oral bioavailability (45%) and is rapidly absorbed (Tmax = 1–1.5 hours) (*Table 4.1*). Rizatriptan is available as 5 mg and 10 mg conventional tablets and as a 10 mg wafer (orally-disintegrating tablet) that dissolves on the tongue. The recommended dose is 10 mg with a maximum of two doses in a 24-hour period.

4.55 What special precautionary measures must be taken with rizatriptan?

Rizatriptan is *contraindicated* for use in patients with ischaemic heart disease, coronary artery disease, Prinzmetal's angina, history of cerebrovascular accident or transient ischaemic attack, peripheral vascular disease, hypertension, basilar or hemiplegic migraine, atypical headache and severe renal or hepatic insufficiency.

Special *precautions* must be taken when rizatriptan is given to patients with risk factors for coronary artery disease or ischaemic heart disease, patients with mild to moderate renal or hepatic insufficiency, those with phenylketonuria (with the ODT formulation, which contains aspartame), the elderly and women who are pregnant or lactating.

Rizatriptan may *interact* with other $5-HT_1$ agonists, ergotamine and its derivatives, MAOIs, propranolol and drugs acting as cytochrome P450 CYP2D6 substrates.

4.56 How effective is oral rizatriptan?

Oral rizatriptan was shown to be significantly superior to placebo for the acute treatment of migraine with an onset of action within 30 minutes of administration. For the conventional tablet, the 5 mg dose is slightly less effective than the 10 mg dose in clinical trials, with 60–63% of patients receiving the 5 mg dose and 67–77% of those receiving the 10 mg dose reporting headache relief 2 hours after treatment (*Table 4.2*).

The conventional tablet formulation of rizatriptan was generally well tolerated in clinical trials. Adverse events that have been reported include dizziness, somnolence, asthenia, abdominal/chest pain, palpitations, tachycardia, gastrointestinal upset, musculoskeletal symptoms, CNS disturbances, pharyngeal discomfort, dyspnoea, pruritus, sweating, urticaria, blurred vision, hot flushes, tongue swelling, rash, toxic epidermal necrolysis and bad sense of taste. Rarely, myocardial ischaemia and infarction, cerebrovascular accidents, syncope and hypertension have been reported.

4.57 How effective is rizatriptan orally-dispersible tablet?

The rizatriptan wafer formulation is rather friable with a mint flavour. It was shown to have a similar clinical profile to the conventional tablet. A total of 66% of patients receiving the 5 mg dose and 74% of those receiving the 10 mg dose reported headache relief at 2 hours (*Table 4.2*).

The ODT formulation of rizatriptan was generally well tolerated in clinical trials and has a tolerability profile similar to the conventional tablet (*see Q 4.56*).

4.58 How does rizatriptan compare with other migraine therapies?

Several studies have shown that rizatriptan is significantly superior to nontriptan acute medications for migraine. Patients reported greater and faster pain relief and a faster resumption of their normal activities following treatment with rizatriptan 5 mg and 10 mg than following the nontriptans.

Rizatriptan may have a slightly faster onset of response and total response than some of the other oral triptans, although the clinical significance of these differences is not clear.

Five controlled clinical trials have compared rizatriptan 10 mg with sumatriptan 25, 50 and 100 mg, naratriptan 2.5 mg and zolmitriptan 2.5 mg. Although rizatriptan was not shown to be significantly superior to the other triptans in terms of the usual primary endpoint in triptan studies (the proportion of patients who reported headache relief at 2 hours), it was significantly superior with respect to certain secondary endpoints for the treatment of moderate to severe headache:

- The proportion of patients pain-free at 2 hours
- The proportion of patients symptom-free at 2 hours
- The proportion of patients with a sustained 24-hour pain-free response
- The proportion of patients who were completely or very satisfied with their treatment.

In four clinical trials comparing rizatriptan with sumatriptan, rizatriptan 10mg had a significantly faster onset of action than sumatriptan 50 mg.

In two preference studies, significantly more patients preferred rizatriptan ODT 10 mg to sumatriptan 50 mg conventional tablets (57% vs 43%, $P < 0.01$ and 64% vs 36%, $P \leq 0.001$).

4.59 How can rizatriptan be recommended as an acute treatment for migraine?

Rizatriptan is an effective and well tolerated acute treatment for migraine. The conventional tablet and ODT oral formulations may have slightly better clinical profiles than at least some of the other oral triptans although the clinical significance of this effect is uncertain. Both oral formulations of rizatriptan can be recommended as first-line acute treatments for migraine. The ODT formulation may be particularly suitable for patients who have unpredictable attacks and need to take their medication at any time or place.

ALMOTRIPTAN

4.60 What are the pharmacological features of almotriptan?

Almotriptan is a highly specific $5\text{-HT}_{1B/1D}$ receptor agonist with a high oral bioavailability (70%), which acts selectively on blood vessels in the brain (*Table 4.1*). It is available as a 12.5 mg conventional tablet. The recommended dose regimen is one tablet, with a maximum of two doses in a 24-hour period.

4.61 What special precautionary measures must be taken with almotriptan?

Almotriptan is *contraindicated* for use in patients with a history or signs of ischaemic heart disease (myocardial infarction, angina, silent ischaemia, Prinzmetal's angina), severe or uncontrolled hypertension, previous cerebrovascular accident, transient ischaemic attack, peripheral vascular disease, severe hepatic impairment and basilar, hemiplegic or ophthalmoplegic migraine.

Special *precautions* must be taken when almotriptan is given to patients with risk factors for underlying cardiovascular disease, patients with severe renal or mild to moderate hepatic impairment, those with a hypersensitivity to sulphonamides, the elderly and women who are pregnant or lactating.

Almotriptan may *interact* with other 5-HT$_1$ agonists, ergotamine and its derivatives and lithium.

4.62 How effective is oral almotriptan?

Oral almotriptan was shown to be significantly superior to placebo for the acute treatment of migraine with an onset of action within 30 minutes of administration. At 2 hours after treatment, between 57–65% of patients receiving almotriptan 12.5 mg reported headache relief (*Table 4.2*). A total of 64% of patients reported headache relief at 2 hours in a meta-analysis of four double-blind, controlled studies. Almotriptan is associated with one of the lowest recurrence rates among the triptans (18–27%).

> Almotriptan was well tolerated in clinical trials with an adverse event profile similar to placebo and few chest symptoms being reported. Reported adverse events included dizziness, somnolence, gastrointestinal upset and fatigue.

4.63 How does almotriptan compare with other migraine therapies?

In a study comparing almotriptan 12.5 mg and sumatriptan 50 mg, similar proportions of patients reported headache relief at 2 hours (58% for almotriptan vs 57% for sumatriptan) and adverse events (15% vs 19%, respectively), although there were significantly fewer chest symptoms in the almotriptan group (<1% vs 2%, $P < 0.01$).

In a second study comparing almotriptan 12.5 mg with sumatriptan 50 mg, patients were equally satisfied with both drugs in terms of the pain relief achieved but were significantly more satisfied with almotriptan in terms of its side effect profile compared with that of sumatriptan ($P = 0.016$).

4.64 How can almotriptan be recommended as an acute treatment for migraine?

Almotriptan is an effective and well tolerated acute treatment for migraine and can be recommended as a first-line acute treatment. Owing to its good safety profile, almotriptan may be suitable as a first-line triptan for patients who are concerned about side effects and as a second-line triptan for those who have experienced worrisome side effects with another triptan. Like naratriptan, almotriptan may also be useful for patients who have reported significant recurrence with other triptans. It is also worth stating that almotriptan is the cheapest of the triptans currently available in the UK.

ELETRIPTAN

4.65 What are the pharmacological features of eletriptan?

Eletriptan is an oral 5-HT$_{1B/1D}$ receptor agonist with high potency and oral bioavailability (50%) which is selective for intracranial blood vessels over extracranial vessels (*Table 4.1*). Eletriptan is the most lipophilic of the available triptans. It is approved as 20, 40 and 80 mg conventional tablets and some doses are marketed in certain countries.

4.66 What special precautionary measures must be taken with eletriptan?

Eletriptan is *contraindicated* for patients with severe renal or hepatic impairment, and for patients aged over 65 years.

Eletriptan should *not be used* together with potent CYP3A4 inhibitors, e.g. erythromycin, clarithromycin and ketoconazole, and protease inhibitors such as ritonavir, indinavir and nelfinavir.

4.67 How effective is oral eletriptan?

Eletriptan was shown to be significantly superior to placebo for the acute treatment of migraine with an onset of action within 30 minutes of administration. In controlled clinical trials, 62–65% of patients receiving eletriptan 40 mg and 65–77% receiving eletriptan 80 mg reported headache relief at 2 hours after treatment (*Table 4.2*).

> Eletriptan is generally well tolerated in clinical studies. The most common side effects reported include asthenia, somnolence, nausea and dizziness.

4.68 How does eletriptan compare with other migraine therapies?

Two clinical trials have demonstrated superior efficacy of eletriptan 40 mg and 80 mg over sumatriptan 50 mg and 100 mg. In the first study, 64% of patients receiving eletriptan 40 mg and 67% receiving 80 mg reported headache relief compared with 50% and 53% receiving sumatriptan 50 mg and 100 mg, respectively. In the second study, the 2-hour headache relief rates were 65% for eletriptan 40 mg, 77% for eletriptan 80 mg and 55% for sumatriptan 100 mg. However these studies have been criticised as the sumatriptan tablets were encapsulated before administration. Encapsulation was shown to delay the absorption of sumatriptan, especially during a migraine attack, which was postulated to account for the relatively low efficacy of the drug in these studies.

4.69 How can eletriptan be recommended as an acute treatment for migraine?

Eletriptan appears to be an effective and well tolerated acute treatment for migraine and will probably become a first-line acute treatment. However, there is very little experience with this drug in clinical practice to date and the true place of eletriptan in migraine therapy will only become clear in the future.

FROVATRIPTAN

4.70 What are the pharmacological features of frovatriptan?

Frovatriptan has a high affinity for the serotonin 5-HT 1B and 1D receptors and is a potent stimulator of vasoconstriction in human basilar arteries. Like naratriptan, it has a long half-life, of 25 hours, but has a relatively low bioavailability (24–30%) (*Table 4.1*). It has been approved for the acute treatment of migraine by the FDA in the USA at an oral dose of 2.5 mg.

4.71 What special precautionary measures must be taken with frovatriptan?

Frovatriptan has not been launched to date and regulatory recommendations for contraindications, special patient populations and drug interactions are not yet available.

4.72 How effective is oral frovatriptan?

Frovatriptan 2.5 mg was shown to be significantly superior to placebo for the acute treatment of migraine but had a slow onset of action (> 2.5 hours). Similar to naratriptan, the headache response following frovatriptan was not optimal at 2 hours after treatment but increased up to 4 hours. In three controlled clinical trials, 36–46% of patients responded to frovatriptan 2.5 mg after 2 hours and 56–65% responded after 4 hours (*Table 4.2*). Interestingly, about one third of patients are reported to respond rapidly to frovatriptan.

> Frovatriptan was generally well tolerated in clinical studies with an adverse event incidence only slightly greater than that reported with placebo. Reported adverse events include dizziness, nausea, headache and fatigue.

4.73 How does frovatriptan compare with other migraine therapies?

No comparative studies have been conducted to date with frovatriptan and other migraine therapies.

4.74 How can frovatriptan be recommended as an acute treatment for migraine?

Frovatriptan appears to be an effective and well tolerated acute treatment for migraine with a clinical profile similar to naratriptan. It is too early to provide recommendations as to its place in therapy, but it is perhaps likely to become a second-line triptan for patients who have tolerability problems with other triptans.

COMPARING THE TRIPTANS

4.75 Is it important to rank the individual drugs within a class?

At the clinical level it may seem unimportant to rank a group of drugs that essentially have the same clinical profile. However, with the triptans there has been intense pressure from the individual manufacturers to attempt to place their triptan in an advantageous position relative to the others. Many claims have been made that may not be justified by the clinical significance of the evidence available. In such a confused area, it is worth evaluating the evidence that compares the triptans in an objective way, to try to provide guidance for the physician.

4.76 How can we understand the evidence used to compare the triptans?

The evidence from clinical studies can be ranked in order of quality, as follows:

- Large, randomised, controlled clinical trials that compare two or more drugs
- Meta-analyses of clinical data
- Smaller randomised studies, open studies and case series
- Post hoc data derived from selected clinical studies
- Consensus agreements between groups of physicians.

The quality of the clinical data comparing the triptans is not optimal. Relatively few large, randomised, controlled trials have compared the clinical profiles of the different triptans and most of these compare the newer oral drugs with the gold standard of oral sumatriptan. One meta-analysis has recently been published that compares the oral triptans. There have also been many post hoc analyses of clinical data which do not provide conclusive evidence of superiority but only suggest future avenues for research. Data analysed in these post hoc analyses include:

- The active response rate (ARR): the proportion of patients reporting headache relief with the triptan
- Placebo response rate (PRR): the proportion of patients reporting headache relief with placebo
- The therapeutic gain (TG): the ARR minus the PRR
- The number needed to treat (NNT): the number of patients it is necessary to treat to achieve one patient with a successful response, adjusted for placebo; this is the reciprocal of the TG.

However, it should be recognised that results from clinical trials do not necessarily equate with those observed in everyday clinical practice. The patients recruited into clinical trials are often not representative of the population with the illness. In the clinic, efficacy rates may be different from those reported in clinical trials and new side effects may emerge following long-term use. The true clinical profile of a drug only reveals itself after extensive use in the clinic.

4.77 How do the triptans rank in terms of clinical profile?

The clinical profiles of the different triptans are summarised in *Table 4.2*. It needs to be recognised that all the triptans are effective and well tolerated acute treatments for moderate to severe migraine. The most effective triptan is subcutaneous sumatriptan 6 mg, which has the greatest 2-hour efficacy and fastest onset of action. Following this, the nasal spray triptans, sumatriptan 20 mg and zolmitriptan 5 mg, have faster onsets of action and possibly slightly greater efficacy than any of the oral formulations.

There seem to be only minor differences in the clinical profile of the oral triptans. The randomised, controlled comparator studies that have been conducted tend to show only small differences between the separate drugs based on secondary endpoints. The meta-analysis of the oral triptans concluded that all available oral triptans are effective and well tolerated acute treatments for migraine but suggested that rizatriptan 10 mg, eletriptan 80 mg and almotriptan 12.5 mg provided the highest likelihood of consistent success. These conclusions have been reinforced by post hoc analyses of selected clinical data and require further investigation in controlled clinical trials. Interestingly, the clinical profiles of the ODT formulations of zolmitriptan and rizatriptan are similar to those of the equivalent conventional tablets.

Patient preference studies provide an alternative means of rating the triptans. In general, they show that individual patients prefer different triptans for their overall effectiveness and speed of effect. However, it is not possible to predict the triptan that the individual patient will prefer.

4.78 Can the oral triptans be differentiated in terms of their clinical profiles?

On the available evidence, the overall ranking of oral triptans has been graded as follows: rizatriptan 10 mg = eletriptan 80 mg > sumatriptan 100 mg = zolmitriptan 2.5 mg > almotriptan 12.5 mg > naratriptan 2.5 mg. However, this needs to be balanced with a consideration of tolerability: adverse events are reported in the rank order eletriptan > zolmitriptan > sumatriptan = rizatriptan > almotriptan > naratriptan. The recently published meta-analysis of all randomised, controlled clinical trials of oral triptans came to the same broad conclusions with rizatriptan 10 mg, eletriptan 80 mg and almotriptan 12.5 mg having the best efficacy profiles.

The overall conclusion that can be made from these studies is that no one oral triptan is substantially superior to another. There is also considerable debate about issues of study design, marketing spin and encapsulation of certain formulations that reduce the clinical utility of the study results. Many headache experts believe that the meta-analysis comparing the triptans is flawed methodologically. Also, the efficacy of a drug as assessed in clinical trials does not necessarily echo its profile in clinical practice. This has been recognised by the FDA, who require the statement 'Comparisons of drug performance based on results obtained in different clinical trials are never reliable' on most triptan labels.

Since patients are treated on an individual basis, the more important question is not which triptan is best relative to another but whether the triptan provided to the patient provides the outcome desired by the patient and healthcare provider. An evaluation of each patient as to their clinical needs and desires should drive the choice of triptan. The factors that should be considered by the physician in prescribing specific triptans are explored in more detail later in this book (*see Qs 5.42–52*).

ERGOTS

4.79 What are the ergots?

> Ergot (*Claviceps purpurea*) is a fungus known since the Middle Ages, when its contamination of wheat led to epidemics of gangrene called 'St Anthony's Fire'. The main causative agent of this is the alkaloid ergotamine. This was isolated in the early part of the 20th century and has been used as an acute treatment for migraine since the 1920s.

4.80 What is the mode of action of the ergots?

The ergots have a complex mechanism of action, involving interactions with several receptors, including alpha-adrenoreceptors, 5-HT and dopamine D_2 receptors.

The mechanism of action of ergotamine and its derivatives in migraine is through a long-acting and nonspecific vasoconstrictor action via 5-HT_1 receptors. This action acts to constrict the cerebral arteries that are dilated during the migraine attack. However, it also acts on cardiac and leg arteries which leads to unwanted side effects.

4.81 What ergot drugs and formulations are available to the physician?

Ergotamine has been used for many years as an acute treatment for moderate to severe migraine, sometimes in combination with caffeine on its own, or the combination of caffeine, pentobarbital and belladonna alkaloids. It can be taken orally, by subcutaneous or intramuscular injection or rectally.

DHE is a derivative of ergotamine that was designed to reduce the incidence of the typical side effects associated with ergotamine. It was developed more recently and clinical studies have used modern criteria for study design, patient selection and methodology. DHE is available by intravenous, subcutaneous and intramuscular injection and as a nasal spray.

ERGOTAMINE

4.82 What special precautionary measures must be taken with ergotamine?

Ergotamine is *contraindicated* for patients with coronary, peripheral or occlusive vascular disease, hypertension, liver or kidney disease, and in women who are pregnant or lactating.

Ergotamine needs to be used with *special care* in patients with infectious hepatitis, sepsis, anaemia and hyperthyroidism.

Ergotamine *cannot* be used with triptans, protease inhibitors, erythromycin, beta-blockers, CNS depressants and alcohol. The dose needs to be reduced if methysergide is being used for migraine prophylaxis.

4.83 How effective are ergotamine-containing products?

Many studies have investigated the clinical profile of ergotamine and its derivatives. However, due to its age these studies often did not use modern dosing strategies and outcome measures. Overall, evidence of ergotamine's efficacy is inconsistent, with some studies finding no effect over placebo and others finding large differences favouring ergotamine.

The oral administration of ergotamine is not optimal due to its very low bioavailability (< 1%). Overall, oral ergotamine does show some superiority over placebo as an acute migraine treatment. However, oral ergotamine was shown to be statistically inferior to oral sumatriptan 100 mg and aspirin plus metoclopramide in controlled clinical studies. Other comparative studies have shown ergotamine to be equivalent to NSAIDs and inferior to isometheptene combinations.

Ergotamine is more bioavailable (1–3%) when given rectally – this is probably the optimal mode of administration for the drug. However, very few studies have been conducted with this formulation. In one double-blind comparator study, ergotamine suppositories (2mg plus 200 mg caffeine) were superior to sumatriptan suppository 25 mg in terms of the proportion of patients reporting headache relief after 2 hours (73% vs 63%). However, more patients preferred sumatriptan (44% vs 36%) due to its better tolerability profile.

> Ergotamine has a suboptimal tolerability profile. Nausea and vomiting are commonly reported as adverse events. Abdominal pain, drowsiness, paraesthesia, swollen fingers and leg cramps may also occur after a single dose. Long-term use is associated with habituation, analgesic rebound headaches, chronic daily headache and leg ischaemia. The clinical use of ergotamine has declined dramatically in recent years and in the UK only the oral combination ergotamine/cyclizine/caffeine product Migril is now available.

4.84 How can ergotamine be recommended as an acute treatment for migraine?

Ergotamine is no longer recommended as an acute treatment for migraine. Compared to the triptans it has suboptimal efficacy and tolerability, together with the risk of serious illness in long-term use. If it has to be used at all, the rectal route should be chosen and the oral route avoided.

DHE

4.85 How does the pharmacology of DHE compare with that of ergotamine?

In general, the pharmacology of DHE is similar to that of ergotamine. DHE is available in parenteral formulations and as a nasal spray. In these formulations, DHE has high bioavailability.

4.86 What special precautionary measures must be taken with DHE?

DHE is *contraindicated* in patients with coronary artery disease, uncontrolled hypertension, known sensitivity to ergot alkaloids, and in pregnant and breast-feeding women.

Although DHE is marketed as an acute treatment for migraine in the USA and many European countries, it is not currently available in the UK.

4.87 How effective is DHE?

Clinical trials have shown that DHE is an effective treatment for moderate to severe migraine. One large, double-blind, controlled clinical study showed that nasal spay DHE 2 mg was significantly superior to placebo as an acute treatment for migraine. At 2 hours after treatment, 65% of patients receiving DHE reported headache relief compared to 23% with placebo ($P < 0.01$). Also, DHE nasal spray was effective in preventing migraine attacks when given during the prodrome phase.

> Although DHE has a better tolerability profile than ergotamine, nausea and vomiting are still frequently reported and co-administration with an antiemetic may be necessary. Other side effects include leg pain and paraesthesia and there are a few reports of angina and ergotism. Additional side effects of transient nasal congestion and throat discomfort are reported with the nasal spray formulation.

4.88 How does DHE compare with other migraine therapies?

Large, controlled, comparator clinical trials have shown that subcutaneous and nasal spray DHE was significantly less effective than subcutaneous sumatriptan. Nasal spray DHE was also significantly less effective than nasal spray sumatriptan. However, the long duration of action of DHE resulted in markedly less headache recurrence than was reported with sumatriptan. The headache relief and recurrence rates reported at 2 hours from these studies are shown in *Table 4.3*.

4.89 How can DHE be recommended as an acute treatment for migraine?

Where they are available, parenteral and nasal spray DHE are effective and reasonably well tolerated acute treatments for migraine. However, the significantly poorer efficacy profile compared to comparable triptan formulations and the potential for safety problems mean that DHE should not be used as a first-line acute treatment. It may be best reserved as a second-line therapy for patients who experience frequent headache recurrences with the triptans.

TABLE 4.3 A comparison of the efficacy of DHE and sumatriptan for the acute treatment of migraine

Study	Dose	Response at 2 hours*	Recurrence rate***
DHE sc	1–2 mg	73%	18%
Sumatriptan sc	6 mg	85%**	45%
DHE in	1–2 mg	53%	17%
Sumatriptan sc	6 mg	81%**	31%
DHE in	1–2 mg	51%	13%
Sumatriptan in	20 mg	63%**	23%

* Proportion of patients reporting an improvement in headache from severe or moderate to mild or none.
** $P < 0.05$
*** Proportion of patients who reported headache relief at 2 hours, but whose headache deteriorated to become severe or moderate at 24 hours after the start of treatment.

ANTIEMETICS

4.90 Are prescription antiemetics effective for migraine?

Antiemetic drugs have been used for the acute treatment of migraine for some time as first-line therapy. However, clinical trials of monotherapy with oral domperidone, prochlorperazine and metoclopramide showed no clinical benefit. However, domperidone and metoclopramide are used together with simple analgesics in combination products which provide effective relief for mild to moderate migraine attacks (*see Q 4.24*).

Parenteral prochlorperazine and metoclopramide have demonstrated some efficacy as acute treatments but are not usually used today as monotherapy for migraine. In some countries they are used as rescue therapy, or as adjuncts to other acute treatments.

Antiemetic drugs are well tolerated by migraine patients, with extrapyramidal side effects (associated with the chronic use of metoclopramide) being reported rarely.
The parenteral antiemetics may be associated with CNS disturbances, anticholinergic effects, sedation, akathisia and ECG and endocrine changes.

CLINICAL PERSPECTIVE ON ACUTE MIGRAINE THERAPIES

4.91 Which of the various acute migraine therapies are effective?

Based on the evidence presented here, the following acute treatments are clinically proven as effective acute treatments for migraine:

■ Aspirin and NSAIDs, used in high doses (e.g. aspirin 900 mg), for mild to moderate attacks
■ Analgesic-antiemetic combination medications, e.g. aspirin plus metoclopramide or paracetamol plus domperidone, for mild to moderate attacks
■ Isometheptene combination medications, for mild to moderate attacks
■ Medications containing opiate analgesics (e.g. codeine), for all attacks
■ Triptans, for all attacks
■ Ergotamine administered rectally, and DHE, for all attacks.

4.92 **Which of the various acute migraine therapies are well tolerated and can be safely administered to patients?**

Based on the evidence presented here, the following acute treatments are clinically proven as well tolerated acute treatments for migraine:

■ Aspirin and NSAIDs, used in high doses (e.g. aspirin 900 mg), for mild to moderate attacks
■ Analgesic-antiemetic combination medications, e.g. aspirin plus metoclopramide or paracetamol plus domperidone, for mild to moderate attacks
■ Isometheptene combination medications, for mild to moderate attacks
■ Triptans, for all attacks.

4.93 **Which of the acute therapies can be recommended for migraine patients?**

Based on the evidence presented here, aspirin and NSAIDs, used in high doses, analgesic-antiemetic combination medications and isometheptene combination medications can be recommended as first-line acute treatments for mild to moderate migraine attacks.
   Triptans are the obvious choice for moderate to severe migraine attacks and for patients who fail on previous therapies. Ergots and preparations containing opiate analgesics should be mostly avoided, except for use as rescue medications and where their use can be monitored.

PROPHYLACTIC TREATMENTS FOR MIGRAINE

4.94 **Which patients should receive prophylaxis for migraine?**

Migraine prophylaxis is worth considering if the patient:

■ Suffers from more than 3–4 attacks per month
■ Experiences significant disability despite receiving acute treatment

■ Suffers from concomitant co-morbidities or a medical illness that precludes effective acute therapy

■ Is at risk of over-using acute medications and therefore developing chronic daily headache

■ Has some of the rare migraine subtypes, such as hemiplegic or basilar migraine, migraine with prolonged aura or migrainous infarction.

However, it should be borne in mind that frequent migraine attacks may also be an indicator for chronic daily headache.

4.95   How do we evaluate the effectiveness of prophylactic treatments for migraine?

Efficacy for prophylactic drugs is defined as a reduction in migraine frequency of > 50%. Although the 'ideal' prophylactic would abolish migraine attacks altogether, in clinical trials only a maximum of about half of patients respond to this extent. Patients therefore need to have an effective acute treatment available for the inevitable breakthrough attacks that occur.

4.96   What are the choices for prophylactic treatments for migraine?

The main prophylactic agents available are beta-blockers, 5-HT$_2$ antagonists, calcium channel antagonists, anticonvulsants and tricyclic antidepressants – although not all of these medications are licensed for migraine in all countries. In recent years the use of migraine prophylaxis has fallen due to the increased availability of effective acute medications, such as the triptans.

BETA-BLOCKERS

4.97   Which beta-blockers are available for migraine prophylaxis?

The noncardioselective beta-blockers propranolol, timolol and nadolol and the cardioselective beta-blockers atenolol and metoprolol have all been used for migraine prophylaxis. Their mechanism of action is probably central in the brain.

4.98   How effective are beta-blockers for preventing migraine?

The beta-blockers propranolol, atenolol, metoprolol, nadolol and timolol have all been shown to be effective in migraine prophylaxis. Placebo-controlled studies showed that propranolol was significantly superior to placebo with 35–60% of patients receiving propranolol reporting ≥ 50% reduction in migraine attack frequency (*Fig. 4.2*). However, propranolol had little effect on reducing the severity or duration of the breakthrough attacks that occurred.

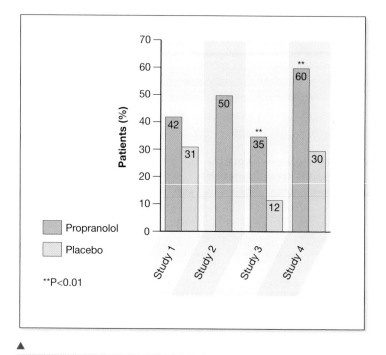

▲

Fig. 4.2 Efficacy of the beta-blocker propranolol for migraine prophylaxis: proportion of patients with a ≥50% reduction in migraine attack frequency.

Other beta-blockers, such as pindolol, alprenolol, oxprenolol and acebutolol, have not been demonstrated to be effective in migraine prophylaxis and are not used in clinical practice.

Due to their effects on the CNS, all beta-blockers can produce behavioural side effects, such as drowsiness, fatigue, lethargy, sleep disorders, nightmares, depression, memory disturbances and hallucinations. Other common side effects include gastrointestinal complaints and decreased exercise tolerance. Less common side effects include orthostatic hypotension, bradycardia, impotence and aggravation of intrinsic muscle disease. Propranolol has been reported to have an adverse effect on the fetus.

Beta-blockers are contraindicated for use in patients with congestive heart failure, asthma and insulin-dependent diabetes. It should also be noted that beta-blockers are banned by international sporting organisations and athletes will be unwilling to take them.

4.99 How can beta-blockers be recommended as prophylaxis for migraine?

The beta-blockers propranolol, atenolol, metoprolol, nadolol and timolol can all be recommended as first-line prophylactic therapy for migraine, although propranolol is usually the agent of choice among them.

SEROTONIN (5-HT₂) ANTAGONISTS

4.100 Which serotonin antagonists are available for migraine prophylaxis?

The serotonin antagonists that have been used for migraine prophylaxis include:

- Pizotifen, a 5-HT_2 receptor antagonist *(not available in the USA)*
- Methysergide, an ergot alkaloid with 5-HT_2 receptor antagonist and $5\text{-HT}_{1B/1D}$ agonist activity
- Cyproheptidine, an antagonist at 5-HT_2, histamine H_1 and muscarinic cholinergic receptors.

4.101 How effective are 5-HT₂ antagonists for preventing migraine?

Pizotifen and methysergide have been shown to be significantly more effective than placebo in migraine prophylaxis. Controlled trials have shown that pizotifen reduces attack frequency by $\geq 50\%$ in 35–50% of patients (*Fig. 4.3*). As with beta-blockers, pizotifen had little effect on the initial severity of breakthrough attacks. Methysergide has been shown to be significantly superior to placebo at reducing headache frequency in four controlled studies. Cyproheptadine appears to be more effective than placebo but less effective than methysergide.

5-HT_2 antagonists are associated with a high frequency of side effects. Pizotifen is associated with drowsiness and increased appetite, which leads to significant weight gain in about 40% of patients. When weight gain occurs, it can limit compliance in what is a primarily female patient population. Pizotifen is contraindicated for breast-feeding women and needs to be used with special care in those with glaucoma, urinary retention, renal impairment and in pregnant women.

Methysergide is associated with transient muscle aching, claudication, abdominal distress, leg cramps, hair loss, nausea, weight gain and hallucinations. Methysergide is contraindicated for patients with peripheral vascular disorders, severe arteriosclerosis, coronary artery disease, valvular heart disease, severe hypertension, thrombophlebitis or cellulitis of the legs, peptic ulcer disease, fibrotic disorders, lung disease, collagen disease, liver or renal impairment, debilitation, serious infections and for pregnant or breast-feeding women.

Cyproheptadine is associated with sedation, weight gain, dry mouth, nausea, light-headedness, ankle oedema, aching legs and diarrhoea. It may also inhibit growth in children. Cyproheptadine is contraindicated in patients with glaucoma, prostatic hypertrophy, bladder neck obstruction, urinary retention, pyoloroduodenal obstruction, stenosing peptic ulcer, acute asthma, elderly debilitated patients, breast-feeding women and neonates.

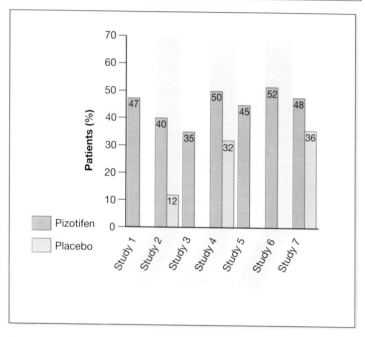

▲

Fig. 4.3 Efficacy of the 5-HT$_2$ antagonist pizotifen for migraine prophylaxis: proportion of patients with a ≥50% reduction in migraine attack frequency.

4.102 How can serotonin antagonists be recommended as prophylaxis for migraine?

The serotonin antagonists pizotifen and methysergide have moderate efficacy in migraine prevention but are associated with too many side effects to be recommended as first-line therapies. They may be used as second-line therapy if other migraine prophylactic drugs are not effective. There is little evidence for the efficacy of cyproheptadine and it cannot be recommended.

CALCIUM CHANNEL ANTAGONISTS

4.103 Which calcium channel antagonists are available for migraine prophylaxis?

The calcium antagonists that have been studied for migraine prophylaxis are flunarizine, verapamil, nifedipine, nimodipine, nicardipine and diltiazem. The mechanism of action of these drugs is unknown but the implication of the calcium channel gene as a possible genetic locus for migraine may be relevant to their activity (*see Q 2.37*).

The availability of calcium channel antagonists for migraine prevention is mixed around the world. No drug in this class is recommended in the UK, flunarizine is available in some European countries but not in the USA – where verapamil can be prescribed.

4.104 How effective are calcium channel antagonists for preventing migraine?

Flunarizine has been shown to be significantly more effective than placebo in over 20 studies in migraine prophylaxis and showed efficacy similar to the beta-blocker metoprolol in one study.

Results for the other calcium channel antagonists are ambiguous. Verapamil, nifedipine, nimodipine, nicardipine and diltiazem either show mixed efficacy in studies or have been investigated to an inadequate extent to arrive at clinical conclusions.

Flunarizine is associated with clinically significant side effects such as sedation, weight gain, abdominal pain, dry mouth, dizziness, hypotension, depression and occasional extrapyramidal symptoms (tremor and Parkinsonism).

Verapamil is also associated with adverse events with constipation being most common, and dizziness, nausea, hypotension, headache and oedema being reported less frequently.

Calcium channel antagonists are contraindicated in patients with congestive heart failure, heart block, hypotension and sick sinus syndrome.

4.105 How can calcium channel antagonists be recommended as prophylaxis for migraine?

Calcium channel blockers have moderate efficacy in migraine prophylaxis but are associated with many side effects. They cannot therefore be recommended as first-line therapies, but, where available, may be used as second-line therapy if other migraine prophylactic drugs have failed.

ANTICONVULSANTS

4.106 Which anticonvulsants are available for migraine prophylaxis?

Anticonvulsants are being increasingly used for migraine prophylaxis, particularly in the USA, although use is mostly off-label elsewhere. They have also proved to be useful in the management of chronic headaches (*see Q 4.127*). The mechanism of action of anticonvulsants in migraine is presumably through pathogenic mechanisms shared by migraine and epilepsy (*see Q 2.11*). The most frequently used anticonvulsant for migraine is sodium valproate or divalproex sodium (an oligomeric complex of sodium valproate and valproic acid). Divalproex sodium is approved for migraine prophylaxis in the USA. Other anticonvulsants investigated for migraine in clinical studies include gabapentin, topiramate, lamotrigine and tiagabine.

4.107 How effective are anticonvulsants for preventing migraine?

Recent clinical trials have shown that sodium valproate and divalproex sodium are effective migraine prophylactic agents with an efficacy profile similar to that of the beta-blockers. Controlled trials have shown that valproate reduced attack frequency by $\geq 50\%$ in 45–50% of patients (*Fig. 4.4*).

Gabapentin has been shown to be moderately effective in a placebo-controlled study in migraine prophylaxis with about one-third of patients having their attack frequency reduced by $\geq 50\%$. An initial placebo-controlled study with topiramate also showed encouraging results with over 45% of patients having their attack frequency reduced by $\geq 50\%$. Both these compounds are now being investigated in large scale, placebo-controlled studies. To date lamotrigine has not demonstrated significant efficacy in migraine and tiagabine has only been investigated in open studies.

Sodium valproate and divalproex sodium were generally well tolerated in clinical studies, the most frequently reported adverse events being mild to moderate nausea, vomiting and gastrointestinal distress. Other adverse events included infection, alopecia, tremor, asthenia, dizziness and somnolence. Rarely, valproate is associated with the severe adverse reactions of hepatitis or pancreatitis. Women of child-bearing potential need to avoid pregnancy while on sodium valproate – it reduces fertility and increases the risk of fetal abnormalities in the first trimester of pregnancy.

Gabapentin is associated with dizziness, giddiness and drowsiness and there is a high incidence of patients withdrawing from therapy. Topiramate is associated with weight loss (rather than with the usual weight gain associated with migraine prophylactics), paraesthesias, somnolence and difficulties with concentration.

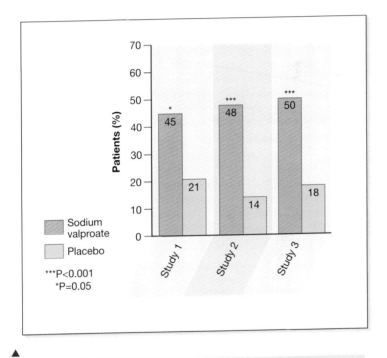

Fig. 4.4 Efficacy of the anticonvulsant sodium valproate for migraine prophylaxis: proportion of patients with a ≥50% reduction in migraine attack frequency.

4.108 How can anticonvulsants be recommended as prophylaxis for migraine?

Sodium valproate / divalproex sodium is clearly an effective migraine prophylactic agent and is generally well tolerated. Where it is licensed for migraine, it is considered a first-line therapy. In other countries it can be considered for off-label use if other prophylactic drugs have failed.

ANTIDEPRESSANTS

4.109 Which antidepressants are available for migraine prophylaxis?

Of the antidepressants, the tricyclics have been used primarily for migraine prophylaxis. Most of the evidence comes from studies with amitriptyline, although dothiepin, nortriptyline and protriptyline have also been investigated. Of the other antidepressants, some studies have investigated the selective serotonin re-uptake inhibitors or SSRIs (e.g. fluoxetine) and others the MAOIs (e.g. phenelzine). The mechanism of action of antidepressants in migraine is unknown but is not the result of treating depression. Antidepressants are useful in treating many chronic pain states, independent of the presence of depression. Antidepressants are not licensed for migraine prophylaxis but are fairly widely used, especially in specialist clinics.

4.110 How effective are antidepressants for preventing migraine?

The antidepressant amitriptyline is used for the prophylaxis of migraine and other headaches, particularly chronic tension-type headache and chronic daily headache (*see Q 4.127*). It is the only antidepressant with reasonably consistent evidence for efficacy in migraine in controlled clinical trials, where it has been shown to be superior to placebo and about as effective as propranolol. It has also proved to be useful in clinical practice. Other tricyclic antidepressants, SSRIs and MAOIs have not been adequately tested for their prophylactic effect in migraine.

> Tricyclic antidepressants are associated with many side effects including sedation, drowsiness, dry mouth, weight gain, constipation, mania, dizziness, tachycardia, blurred vision, tremor, confusion, arterial hypotension, urinary retention and akathesia. Amitriptyline and doxepin are markedly sedating, nortriptyline and protriptyline less so.

4.111 How can antidepressants be recommended as prophylaxis for migraine?

Amitriptyline is an effective migraine prophylactic agent but has tolerability problems that can restrict its general use. As it is not licensed for migraine, its use should probably be restricted to secondary care. However, it may be considered for first-line use if the patient has depression as well as migraine.

4.112 What other prophylactic drugs are used to treat migraine?

In some countries, aspirin and other NSAIDs and DHE are used to treat migraine prophylactically, although they are not licensed for this use in the

UK and the USA. Aspirin and NSAIDs (especially naproxen) have some evidence of efficacy in migraine prophylaxis, although their gastrointestinal side effects limit the chronic use of these drugs. COX-2 inhibitors may have greater clinical potential due to their lower potential to cause gastrointestinal irritation. DHE is used as a prophylactic in certain European countries even though there are few clinical data to support its use. Also, daily use of DHE can lead to the development of chronic daily headache and ergotism. The lack of proven efficacy for these compounds and their known risk of significant side effects mean that they cannot be recommended for use in migraine prophylaxis.

Several new drug therapies are currently in development or have shown some evidence of effect for the prophylaxis of migraine and other headaches. These include Botulinum toxin type A (Botox), montelukast and tizanidine – these drugs are discussed later (*see Q 8.12*).

In addition, vitamins (e.g. riboflavin [B2]), minerals (e.g. magnesium) and herbs (e.g. feverfew) have all been studied for migraine prophylaxis, and feverfew is widely used by migraine sufferers. These compounds are considered below (Alternative therapies for migraine).

4.113 Which of the migraine prophylactic drugs can be recommended as first-line therapy?

Drugs with proven efficacy for migraine prophylaxis that can be used as first-line therapies include:

■ The beta-blockers propranolol, timolol and metoprolol
■ The calcium antagonist flunarizine
■ The anticonvulsant sodium valproate / divalproex sodium
■ The antidepressant amitriptyline.

Drugs that may be effective, but without large double-blind, placebo-controlled clinical trials demonstrating their efficacy, or that have serious side effects that limit their use include:

■ The 5-HT$_2$ antagonists pizotifen and methysergide
■ Other anticonvulsants and antidepressants
■ DHE
■ Aspirin and NSAIDs.

ALTERNATIVE THERAPIES FOR MIGRAINE

4.114 Why do migraine sufferers want alternative therapies for migraine?

Many migraine sufferers are attracted to alternative treatments for their migraine, for a variety of reasons:

■ They have exhausted all conventional options
■ They feel it is a fashionable option
■ The therapist gives them more time than their physician does
■ They feel that these therapies offer them a greater level of individual control
■ They assume that alternative therapies are more 'natural' and safe.

4.115 What alternative therapies have been tried for migraine?

Alternative treatments used fall into two categories – prophylactic therapies and lifestyle changes. Treatments that sufferers can buy OTC in pharmacists or in health food shops in an attempt to reduce the frequency of their migraine headaches include feverfew, homeopathic remedies, riboflavin and magnesium. Some patients try the nonpharmacological intervention of acupuncture. Aromatherapy, dietary therapies and the limiting of foods thought to cause 'allergies' or 'intolerances' are all used by some migraine sufferers.

4.116 Is there clinical evidence for the use of feverfew for migraine?

Three clinical studies have indicated that feverfew (*Tanacetum parthenium*) may be effective as migraine prophylaxis. One study showed a reduction in attack frequency and severity with feverfew compared with placebo. A second study showed an increase in the frequency and severity of attacks when feverfew treatment was stopped in patients taking the treatment. The third study indicated that feverfew use led to significant reductions in headache, nausea, vomiting, photophobia and phonophobia compared to placebo. However, a fourth study showed no difference between feverfew and placebo. Feverfew may therefore be useful for migraine prophylaxis but should be used with caution, as its safety profile has not been evaluated in controlled clinical trials and commercial preparations differ widely in the concentration of active ingredient. Reported side effects include mouth ulceration and a more widespread oral inflammation associated with loss of taste.

There is also a feverfew nasal spray available now for the acute treatment of migraine although there seems to be no clinical evidence of its efficacy and tolerability.

4.117 Is there clinical evidence for the use of homeopathic remedies for migraine?

Evidence for the utility of homeopathic remedies in migraine is limited to two conflicting clinical trials. One randomised, double-blind study indicated that homeopathic treatment was no better than placebo. The second study, although showing that homeopathic medications reduced the frequency of migraine attacks, did not select migraine patients on the basis of the IHS diagnostic criteria – which raises questions as to the validity of the patient population studied. Based on these results, homeopathic remedies cannot be recommended for the prophylaxis of migraine.

4.118 Is there clinical evidence for the use of riboflavin for migraine?

Compared to people without migraine, the brain of migraine sufferers may have a mitochondrial dysfunction resulting in impaired oxygen metabolism. The rationale for using riboflavin as a migraine prophylactic agent is that it has the potential to increase mitochondrial energy efficiency. A single controlled clinical trial has shown that high-dose riboflavin was significantly more effective than placebo in migraine prophylaxis. Riboflavin reduced attack frequency by $\geq 50\%$ in 59% of patients compared with 15% for placebo ($P < 0.01$) and was well tolerated. However, further studies are required to confirm these data before riboflavin can be unhesitatingly recommended for clinical use.

4.119 Is there clinical evidence for the use of magnesium for migraine?

Brain magnesium levels are low during the migraine attack which may affect migraine-related receptors and neurotransmitters. The daily supplementation of magnesium can theoretically replace this magnesium and therefore prevent migraine attacks. Two controlled clinical trials have shown that chronic oral supplementation of magnesium significantly reduced the frequency of migraine attacks compared with placebo. However, a third study showed no benefit over placebo in terms of reducing attack frequency by $\geq 50\%$, the recognised standard for efficacy. More studies are therefore required before magnesium can be added to the armamentarium of clinically-proven migraine prophylactic agents.

4.120 Is there clinical evidence for the use of acupuncture for migraine?

A systematic, evidence-based review has recently been published on the effectiveness of acupuncture in primary headaches. Of the 16 trials comparing true acupuncture with 'sham' acupuncture in migraine and tension-type headache:

- Eight trials showed true acupuncture to be significantly superior
- Four trials showed a trend in favour of true acupuncture
- Two trials showed no difference between the treatments
- Two trials were not interpretable.

This evidence supports the value of acupuncture as a treatment for migraine and tension-type headache. However, larger and more rigorous trials are required to determine the true place of acupuncture in migraine therapy.

4.121 Is there clinical evidence for the use of aromatherapy for migraine?

Although many complementary and alternative medicine practitioners advocate aromatherapy for migraine, there is no objective clinical evidence for its efficacy. However, it is plausible that it could inhibit the development of migraine attacks by reducing stress and there are unlikely to be any side effects.

4.122 Is there clinical evidence for the use of food allergy testing for migraine?

A few physicians believe that migraine is an atopic disorder and that migraine attacks may correlate with increased histamine levels. Certain foods are proposed to provoke migraine attacks by increasing IgE and histamine levels. A few small studies, particularly in children, have indicated that therapy using drugs or diet restrictions could reduce the incidence of migraine headaches. In addition, food intolerances have been linked to migraine through a proposed weakening of the immune system via IgG mechanisms. Kits for testing for food intolerances are available commercially. If the patient exhibits an IgG response to specific foods, it is proposed that this be used as a starting point for further investigations and/or the introduction of exclusion diets.

The linkage of foods to migraine has always been a tangled web, due also to the proposed existence of food trigger factors (*see Q 2.48*). The concept that migraine may be due to food allergies and/or intolerances is highly controversial and mostly based on anecdotal evidence. Evidence from large, randomised placebo-controlled studies is required before any link between migraine and food allergy or intolerance can be substantiated.

4.123 Can any alternative therapies be recommended for migraine treatment?

Of the alternative therapies evaluated for migraine, the following have clinical evidence of efficacy and may therefore be recommended by the physician:

- Feverfew prophylaxis
- Magnesium prophylaxis
- Riboflavin prophylaxis
- Acupuncture prophylaxis.

The patient needs to decide which, if any, of these therapies appeals to them, is affordable or practicable to their lifestyles. In addition, alternative stress reduction strategies, such as aromatherapy, reflexology or yoga, may all be beneficial.

TREATMENTS FOR OTHER HEADACHE TYPES

4.124 What treatments have been assessed for tension-type headache?

Since acute tension-type headache produces little impact and is readily managed by most people outside the healthcare system, it is not commonly encountered on its own in medical practice. It is, however, frequently seen as part of the headache spectrum in those with migraine. In this setting, based on its response to triptans, many physicians consider it to have a similar pathophysiology to migraine. In fact, it has been suggested that tension-type headache in migraine sufferers is a distinct entity from tension-type headache without migraine.

Management of acute tension-type headache usually includes OTC medications such as aspirin, paracetamol and NSAIDs and nondrug approaches such as relaxation, hot baths and massage. These treatments are usually effective and further intervention is rarely necessary. Management of chronic tension-type headache is more complex and is dealt with below (*see* Q *4.127*) but amitriptyline has been shown to be effective as prophylaxis. Amitriptyline tends to be used as, unlike dothiepin, it has no associated risk for developing ischaemic heart disease.

4.125 What treatments have been assessed for short, sharp headache?

Owing to the short duration of these headaches, acute treatments tend to be of little use and reassurance that these headaches are benign is usually enough to satisfy the patient. However, various prophylactic medications can be useful:

- NSAIDs taken daily, e.g. diclofenac or indomethacin
- Valproate
- Tricyclic antidepressants, which are also used for chronic paroxysmal hemicrania.

4.126 What treatments have been assessed for cluster headache?

Cluster headaches are usually managed by neurologists or headache specialists in the secondary care setting. Since cluster headaches are of short duration, abortive treatment must be rapid in onset and thus oral formulations are of limited value. Successfully used drugs include the following:

■ Subcutaneous sumatriptan 6 mg is very effective against cluster headache and is the abortive treatment of choice. Nasal spray sumatriptan 20 mg is also effective. However, oral triptans are relatively ineffective. Oral zolmitriptan 5 mg has only modest efficacy against episodic cluster headache, much lower than subcutaneous sumatriptan or oxygen.

■ Inhalation of high flow-rate oxygen is also effective as an abortive treatment in about 70% of patients, usually within 5–10 minutes of dosing.

■ Nasally-applied lignocaine is a useful adjunct to other abortive therapies.

Prophylaxis is the mainstay of cluster headache management, initiated at the beginning of a new cluster period. The following drugs have been shown to be effective:

■ Corticosteroids (prednisolone), methysergide and ergotamine can be used for short-term prophylaxis. Prednisolone can provide relief for chronic cluster attacks or cover the introduction of medication at the beginning of a cluster period.

■ Verapamil and lithium are used for long-term prophylaxis.

4.127 What treatments have been assessed for chronic daily headache?

Cases of chronic daily headache are usually referred to neurologists or headache specialists for management. There are four strategies for the management of this headache:

1. Physical measures, such as physiotherapy of the neck. This is of help when the patient, as often occurs, has a history of head or neck injury.
2. Withdrawal of drugs causing rebound headaches, such as codeine and ergotamine.
3. Headache prophylactic drugs, including:
   ■ Tricyclic antidepressants, e.g. prothiaden and amitriptyline.
   ■ Anticonvulsants, e.g. valproate, gabapentin and topiramate.
4. Acute medications to treat breakthrough migraine attacks, e.g. triptans.

4.128 What treatments have been assessed for sinus headache?

First-line therapy for sinus headaches of infectious aetiology is:

■ A broad-spectrum antibiotic
■ Local measures, e.g. steam inhalation or vasoconstrictor agents
■ Oral decongestants, if treatment is required for more than 72 hours

If this fails, referral to a specialist is probably required.

4.129 What treatments have been assessed for other types of facial pain?

Trigeminal neuralgia: The first-line drug for trigeminal neuralgia is usually the anticonvulsant carbamazepine. Alternatives include other anticonvulsants (valproate or gabapentin), the muscle relaxant baclofen and the benzodiazepine clonazepam. The patient can be referred for surgery if these drugs do not control the symptoms.

Postherpetic neuralgia: Three strategies are used in series to manage this condition, dependent on the stage of the illness:

■ During the acute eruption of pain, the best approach is the use of antiviral drugs such as aciclovir or valaciclovir. There is a greatly reduced likelihood of patients developing postherpetic pain if they take these drugs very early in the illness.

■ In the acute phase of the rash, analgesics are often used, together with topical applications such as camomile to reduce local irritation.

■ Once the rash has cleared and a definite diagnosis of herpetic neuralgia made, tricyclic antidepressants are the mainstay of treatment, together with local application of capsaicin.

Temporomandibular joint dysfunction: This condition is usually managed by a dentist, e.g. by fitting a customised gum shield for use at night. Supplementary medical strategies include stress management programmes and prophylaxis with tricyclic antidepressants.

4.130 What drugs will I need for my migraine?

Almost all migraine sufferers use some kind of medication to treat their attacks. Medications include those used to stop an existing attack (acute medications) and those used to prevent attacks occurring (prophylactic medications).

Every migraine sufferer needs acute medications to treat attacks when they occur. The range of acute medications available is wide and includes a variety of prescription and over-the-counter pain medications, prescription medications for nausea and prescription medications specifically for migraine – which are the most effective therapies. Prescription medications may be in the form of tablets, nasal sprays or injections. Many patients use more than one type of medication or combinations of these products to treat the various presentations of migraine they experience. The most important attribute of a medication for treating migraine is that it safely and consistently puts a stop to the migraine symptoms.

There is also a range of prophylactic medications available. Most are prescription medications but the herb feverfew, acupuncture, biofeedback and relaxation, and stress reduction techniques may also prevent migraine when used on a regular basis.

4.131 Does nondrug therapy work for migraine?

Nondrug therapies are valuable approaches to migraine treatment, usually taken together with prophylactic and/or acute drugs. The therapies with the best chances of success are biofeedback, relaxation training and stress reduction strategies. These therapies help to prevent migraine attacks developing and there is nothing to stop you trying two or more of them at the same time. However, they do not stop migraine attacks altogether and it is important to keep on taking your prescribed medications.

Note: Biofeedback is training the body to bring involuntary physiological functions under voluntary control. Biofeedback trains the nervous system to shut out excessive stimulation through calming music, visualisation and slow diaphragmatic breathing. Biofeedback is usually obtained through practitioners of complementary medicine, although it is possible to train yourself with self-help books.

4.132 Do aspirin and paracetamol work for migraine?

Aspirin and other nonsteroidal anti-inflammatory drugs (NSAIDs) such as ibuprofen can work as acute treatments for migraine but may need to be taken in larger doses than normal to be effective. If you find that two aspirins or ibuprofens do not work for migraine, it is best to see your doctor for advice. Unfortunately, paracetamol does not work for migraine and should not be used on its own. You can buy drug combinations of paracetamol and codeine at your pharmacist. These are quite effective for migraine but should not be used regularly. If you find that you need to take them on more than two days per week, you should go to see your doctor for advice.

4.133 What are the combination analgesics?

Sometimes painkillers such as aspirin and paracetamol are combined with other drugs to make them work better on migraine. These extra drugs are usually antiemetics, to prevent the sick feelings associated with migraine. The combination analgesics are only available from your doctor with a prescription.

4.134 What are triptan drugs?

Triptans are a class of acute medications that are designed specifically to treat attacks of migraine. They are chemically designed to mimic serotonin, a chemical used by nerves to communicate with each other. Serotonin levels are low during migraine and triptan drugs assist the nervous system with re-establishing control of function. There are several triptans that are currently available and although they differ slightly in their chemical characteristics, they all function in the same way.

4.135 How do triptans work?

Migraine is a complex process that can affect the body in many ways. During migraine attacks blood vessels around the brain can swell and become inflamed. As this happens, the nervous system's ability to block pain is decreased. Triptans work by decreasing the swelling of the blood vessels and the inflammation of nerves involved in the migraine process. They also restore the nervous system's ability to block pain impulses. This is why they are considered to be migraine-specific medications.

4.136 How effective are the triptans?

The triptans are the best available acute treatments for migraine and most people who take them obtain effective relief of their migraines, usually within 2 hours of taking the pill. The different triptans are available in different forms: ordinary tablets, tablets that dissolve on the tongue without water, nasal sprays and injections that you can do yourself.

4.137 Is it safe to take triptans?

Triptans are one of the most thoroughly studied drugs ever. They have been used by millions of migraine sufferers and for literally hundreds of millions of migraine attacks. They have an excellent overall safety profile. However, as with all medications, they are not perfect. There have been rare reports of heart problems associated with triptan use. It is therefore important to discuss your risk for heart disease with your doctor. In addition, there are certain medications that should not be taken with a triptan drug and there are specific types of headaches for which a triptan should not be given. These issues too should be discussed with your doctor.

4.138 I've used ergotamine in the past. Is it OK to go on using it?

Ergotamine is a rather old-fashioned drug now and has been generally superseded by the triptans. It is not as effective as the triptans and has a lot more side effects. These days, ergotamine is only used for patients with infrequent migraines or those where the headaches last a long time. You should never use ergotamine on a regular basis. You should go to see your doctor if you are taking ergotamine on more than a couple of occasions per month.

4.139 When do you need to take prophylactic medications for migraine?

You will probably need to take a prophylactic medication when you get more than three or four migraine attacks every month, or if acute medications don't work or cause a lot of side effects. Some people prefer to take a pill every day to try to stop attacks occurring. However, do remember that prophylactic medications do not stop all migraine attacks and you also need an acute medication to treat the attacks that do occur.

4.140 What prophylactic medications am I likely to be given?

You are most likely to be first given a drug called a beta-blocker for migraine prophylaxis. This is usually effective, but might cause some side effects such as drowsiness, sleep problems, memory problems and depression. You should not take these drugs if you are a competitive athlete, as they are banned by the Olympics and other sporting bodies.

If the beta-blocker does not work, or you can't stand the side effects, you may be given another drug. This might be an antidepressant or antiepilepsy drug. Don't worry, these drugs also work for migraine and don't mean you have the other illness. You might also be given a serotonin antagonist. These are quite effective but do cause a lot of side effects. They can cause quite a lot of weight gain, so you should be prepared for this before you take them. The serotonin antagonist pizotifen (Sanomigran) is often used as a first-line treatment for migraine in the UK, so you might be offered this first.

4.141 Can I try herbal remedies or acupuncture for migraine prophylaxis?

Small studies have shown that feverfew (obtainable from your pharmacist or from health food shops) can prevent migraine attacks from occurring in some cases and you might find it useful. Some studies have also shown that riboflavin (Vitamin B2) and magnesium may be effective. These are also easily available from pharmacists and health food shops and may be worth a try. Acupuncture seems to work for some sufferers as migraine prophylaxis, although it does not work for everyone and may cause unacceptable pain and discomfort to some.

At the end of the day, it is your decision as to which alternative therapies to try. They tend to work for some people but not for others. There are few scientific studies to base a decision on. From a practical standpoint, the real question is, can these treatments help you? From that perspective, you can try these treatments and see if they work for you.

4.142 What is the best way to treat tension-type headache?

Treatment for tension-type headache is best determined by the circumstances that accompany the headache. If tension-type headache is isolated and the only type of headache a person experiences, it may be treated with rest, sleep, exercise, or possibly a simple nonprescription painkiller. If tension-type headaches are frequent, then preventative medications are recommended and you should see your doctor for treatment. If tension headache is often a harbinger to migraine then it should be treated as migraine. If tension-type headache is a component of chronic daily headache then treatment needs to be coordinated by your doctor.

Management of migraine in clinical practice

5

CHOOSING THE OPTIMAL PROPHYLACTIC THERAPY

FOLLOW-UP CONSULTATIONS

MIGRAINE MANAGEMENT IN PRIMARY CARE TODAY

5.1 What healthcare providers do migraine sufferers use the most?

The majority of headache management takes place in the primary care setting. Over 90% of headache cases in the UK and over 50% of migraine cases in Denmark, the Netherlands, Canada and the USA are dealt with initially by primary care physicians. Only a minority of cases need referral to a specialist. Other healthcare providers used by migraine patients as their initial point of contact include:

■ Specialists, used by a minority of patients almost solely in the USA and Canada, include neurologists, gynaecologists, obstetricians, ophthalmologists and pain and headache specialists
■ Hospital emergency rooms, again used significantly only in North America by a minority of patients, often for rescue therapy
■ Alternative practitioners, e.g. physiotherapists, homeopaths and acupuncturists, used by a significant minority of patients in the USA and Europe
■ Pharmacists, used by most headache sufferers and solely relied on by about 15% of sufferers internationally.

5.2 What current guidelines do physicians have for the management of migraine?

Management guidelines for migraine have been published in many countries, including the UK, USA and Germany. These guidelines, while comprehensive, are perhaps better suited for specialist use than in primary care. They tend to emphasise a rigorous diagnostic procedure followed by the inefficient step-wise approach to care (see Q 4.5). These guidelines require a significant investment in time and effort for the physician and the patient with no guarantee of success in the short term. There is another, more subtle point, which can be described as 'medicine is the art of the possible'. After years of promotion of these types of guideline, there have been no major inroads into the way many primary care physicians manage headache. The inescapable conclusion is that this recommended approach does not seem worthwhile to primary care physicians. There is a wide gap between what often happens in primary care practice and what specialists are recommending, the end result being the poor consultation, diagnostic and treatment success rates seen for migraine.

5.3 How well is migraine managed in primary care today?

Even though migraine is a significant personal and public health problem, it is not always managed effectively in primary care. Less than 50% of migraine sufferers receive effective treatment from their healthcare providers. This is largely due to variability of the condition on presentation.

The problems associated with migraine care can perhaps best be understood as a series of barriers that the patient has to overcome before they receive effective care (*Fig. 5.1*):

■ Over half of migraine patients do not consult their primary care physician for medical care
■ Only about half of primary care physicians seem able to diagnose migraine in a presenting patient
■ Despite the proven effectiveness of migraine-specific medications, the majority of migraine sufferers rely on suboptimal over-the-counter (OTC) medications

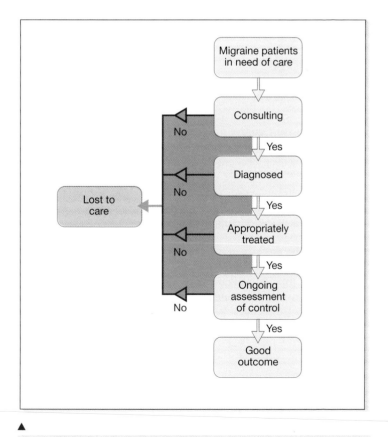

▲
Fig. 5.1 Barriers to migraine care in clinical practice.

■ Follow-up of migraine care is poor, with many patients lapsing from care before receiving effective treatment.

5.4 How many migraine sufferers consult their primary care physician for care?

The majority of migraine sufferers worldwide do not currently consult their physicians about the condition (*Table 5.1*). A substantial proportion has never seen a physician about migraine. Nevertheless, many people who never consult suffer significantly from their migraine. In one study, 60% of nonconsulting American women reported severe to very severe pain and 68% reported severe disability or were forced to rest in bed during their attacks. Of sufferers who do consult a physician, the pattern seems to be an initial consultation period of about 1 year, followed by a lapse in care-seeking behaviour thereafter.

The main reasons given by migraine sufferers for not consulting include:

■ A belief that there is nothing the physician can do to help
■ Dissatisfaction with the care received from their physicians.

5.5 How well do primary care physicians diagnose migraine?

Studies conducted in primary care in the USA and France showed that over half of migraine sufferers who consulted for headache (55% in the USA and 58% in France) did not receive an accurate diagnosis from their physician. In the UK, only 2% of consulting patients in two general practices had received a diagnosis of migraine in the previous 5 years, whereas the expected figure from the known migraine prevalence should have been about 10%. Patients who tended not to be diagnosed were:

TABLE 5.1 Consultation patterns for migraine. Results from population-based epidemiological studies

Study country and date	Proportion of patients (%)			
	Ever consulted	Current consulter	Lapsed consulter	Never consulted
UK, 1999	86	49	37	14
Canada, 1993	81	36	45	19
USA, 1998	67	47	21	32
International*, 1993	66	31	35	34
Denmark, 1992	56	ND	ND	44
Japan, 1997	31	15	16	69

* Study conducted in Belgium, Canada, Italy, Sweden and the UK
ND = No data

- Men
- Those with migraine without aura
- Those with depression as well as migraine
- Those without significant headache-related disability.

5.6 How well are migraine patients treated by their primary care physicians?

Although many effective treatments are now available for migraine, the sufferer who consults a physician and receives an accurate diagnosis may still not receive appropriate therapy. Most migraine sufferers in Europe and North America rely on OTC medications, relatively few taking prescription drugs (*Table 5.2*).

Furthermore, many migraine sufferers do not report effective relief with their antimigraine medications. In the USA, only 29% of migraine sufferers stated that they were satisfied with their usual acute treatments. Features that led to dissatisfaction included:

- A lack of overall relief
- Delay in the onset of relief
- Too many side effects.

5.7 How has medical care for migraine changed over the last decade?

The under-consultation, under-diagnosis and under-treatment of migraine have continued with only minor improvements over the past decade. The irony is that, during this time period, new, effective migraine therapies have become available and the physician has never had more to offer the patient.

Comparing two identical epidemiological studies conducted in the USA in 1989 and 1998, the proportion of migraine sufferers consulting their

---

TABLE 5.2 Proportion of migraine sufferers using prescription and OTC medications

Study country and date	Sufferers (%)		
	Prescription medications	OTC medications	No medications
International**, 1999	45*	58*	11
Canada, 1993	44*	91*	ND
USA, 1989	37	59	4

* Some sufferers took both prescription and OTC medications
** Study conducted in France, Germany, Italy, Sweden, UK, Canada and USA
ND = No data

> **TABLE 5.3 Comparison of migraine consultation and diagnostic rates, and use of prescription medications, in two US studies conducted in 1989 and 1998**
>
> | | Proportion of sufferers | |
> | --- | --- | --- |
> | | 1989 | 1998 |
> | Migraine sufferers consulting with their physicians | 16% | 48% |
> | Physician diagnosis of migraine | 38% | 48% |
> | Migraine patients using prescription drugs | 37% | 41% |

physicians increased three-fold, but is still presently less than 50%, while the increase in the rate of physician diagnosis and use of prescription therapies has been disappointingly low (*Table 5.3*).

PRINCIPLES FOR IMPROVING MIGRAINE MANAGEMENT IN PRIMARY CARE

5.8   What is the prognosis for migraine?

Migraine is essentially an illness of young and middle-aged people; people completing their education, beginning and developing their careers, raising their children and starting to look after aged relatives. People, therefore, who can least afford to have such a painful, disabling and unpredictable condition.

However, the prognosis for migraine should be good. It is a self-limiting condition, which although not curable, is usually manageable to an extent that sufferers can work and function reasonably normally, even during their attacks. The challenge for physicians is to improve current management practices, to provide effective treatment and so improve the prognosis.

5.9   What are the current unmet needs of migraine sufferers?

Migraine sufferers differ in their management needs, largely due to the variation in severity of symptoms and their impact on the sufferer. Although severely affected sufferers tend to receive more medical care than those less affected, a significant proportion of those with severe pain and disability remain undetected, undiagnosed and under-treated in clinical practice. Initiatives are needed to improve migraine care in several areas to provide a service focused on the individual patient's needs.

5.10   What should the physician's goals be to improve migraine management?

As primary care physicians are the medical service most commonly used by migraine sufferers, it makes sense to coordinate headache management services around them. Unfortunately, the education of primary care physicians about headache is usually limited to the exclusion of serious but rare secondary (sinister) headaches rather than the management of the common benign primary headaches. Primary care physicians also have severe limitations to the time they can give each patient. Simple, clear and unified guidelines are therefore needed to allow the primary care physician to deal with patients with headache. The overall goals should be to:

- Accurately diagnose and provide appropriate treatment for the majority of patients who can be managed in primary care
- Rapidly identify and refer the minority of patients who need to be seen by a specialist.

The means to achieve these goals are as follows:

- Encourage migraine sufferers to engage with the healthcare system, to consult their primary care provider and receive appropriate treatment
- Motivate currently consulting migraine patients to continue with their care
- Provide physicians with simple but comprehensive guidelines to allow them to diagnose migraine differentially from other headaches
- Encourage physicians to provide prescription medications that have been proven to be effective.

PROVIDING NEW GUIDELINES FOR MIGRAINE MANAGEMENT

5.11 What new guidelines are available for migraine management in primary care?

Recently, several initiatives have been undertaken to develop new guidelines for the management of migraine in primary care, including those issued by the Migraine in Primary Care Advisors (MIPCA) in the UK and the Headache Consortium and the Primary Care Network in the USA.

5.12 What are the guidelines of the Migraine in Primary Care Advisors?

MIPCA guidelines were first issued in 1997 and revised guidelines were published in 2000. MIPCA advocates an individualised approach to care, treatment being prescribed according to each patient's needs. Factors considered include the nature of the patient's attacks, the impact of headache on the individual's life and the demands of the patient's lifestyle (*Fig. 5.2*).

At the initial consultation, the physician is recommended to conduct a diagnostic assessment and to take a careful history covering the nature of the headaches, previous treatments taken and the impact on the patient's

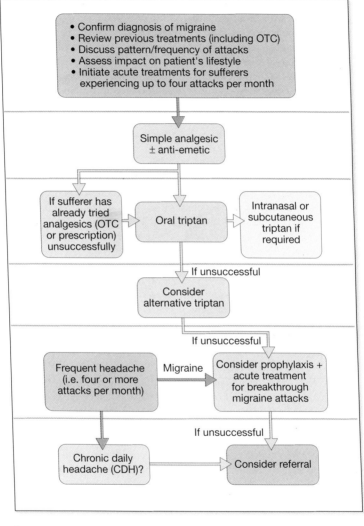

Fig. 5.2 The 2000 MIPCA guidelines for headache management.

life. Patients who experience up to four attacks per month are given acute therapy with a simple analgesic (with or without an antiemetic) or an oral triptan if analgesics have been used unsuccessfully in the past. Nasal spray or subcutaneous triptan formulations may be considered if the patient has difficulties with oral therapies or requires a fast therapeutic effect due to the demands of their lifestyle or presentation characteristics of their headaches.

It is essential to establish a goal for therapeutic intervention. Useful goals centre on preservation of function or being free of pain and associated migraine symptoms. Merely providing enough relief to 'get through' an attack commonly results in the patients lapsing from care.

If the initial therapy is unsuccessful, an alternative triptan may be provided. For patients who fail on this therapy, and for migraine patients with four or more headaches per month, prophylactic treatment is recommended with additional acute treatment for breakthrough attacks. Migraine patients who fail on this treatment, and those diagnosed with chronic daily headache, may require referral to a specialist physician.

The MIPCA guidelines have been recently under review and new guidelines were published during the latter half of 2002.

5.13 What are the US Headache Consortium Guidelines?

New practice guidelines for the management of migraine were published by the US Headache Consortium in 2000. Identified goals of successful migraine management were reduction of attack frequency, severity and disability, improvement of quality of life, prevention of headache, avoidance of the escalation of acute medications and the education of patients to better self-manage their illness.

The US Headache Consortium identified several principles of managing migraine (*Fig. 5.3*). Following a diagnostic assessment, the physician is recommended to assess the illness severity, by taking a history of attack frequency and severity, degree of disability, the presence of nonheadache symptoms and patient-specific factors such as their prior response to medications and coexistent conditions. A major part of these guidelines is the education of patients about their condition and its treatment, to establish realistic expectations and to encourage them to participate in the management of their migraine. Finally, an individualised treatment plan is advocated, tailoring therapy to the patient's symptoms, illness severity, disability and personal needs.

The US Headache Consortium mostly used evidence-based medicine to rate different treatments but where this was not possible due to lack of data, a consensus was reached. They recommend a stratified approach to care (*see Q 4.7*), whereby the initial prescribed therapy is based on a baseline assessment of the illness severity and treatment needs of the patient. Nonsteroidal anti-inflammatory drugs (NSAIDs and combinations of

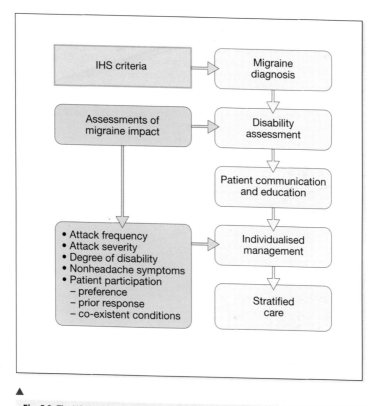

Fig. 5.3 The US Headache Consortium Guidelines for migraine management.

analgesics with antiemetics are recommended for patients with mild to moderate migraine. Migraine-specific agents (e.g. triptans) are recommended for patients with moderate to severe migraine and for those who have previously failed on the NSAIDs and combination analgesics. The consortium advocates a nonoral route of administration for patients with severe nausea and vomiting and a rescue medication for treatment failures. Finally, physicians are cautioned to guard against the overuse of headache medications.

5.14 What are the US Primary Care Network guidelines?

The Primary Care Network is a group of physicians working in private practice, managed care and academia, who provide medical programmes for the management of diseases in US primary care. They published a

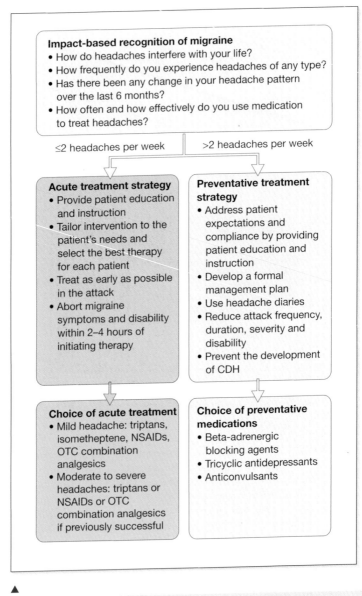

Impact-based recognition of migraine
- How do headaches interfere with your life?
- How frequently do you experience headaches of any type?
- Has there been any change in your headache pattern over the last 6 months?
- How often and how effectively do you use medication to treat headaches?

≤2 headaches per week   >2 headaches per week

Acute treatment strategy
- Provide patient education and instruction
- Tailor intervention to the patient's needs and select the best therapy for each patient
- Treat as early as possible in the attack
- Abort migraine symptoms and disability within 2–4 hours of initiating therapy

Preventative treatment strategy
- Address patient expectations and compliance by providing patient education and instruction
- Develop a formal management plan
- Use headache diaries
- Reduce attack frequency, duration, severity and disability
- Prevent the development of CDH

Choice of acute treatment
- Mild headache: triptans, isometheptene, NSAIDs, OTC combination analgesics
- Moderate to severe headaches: triptans or NSAIDs or OTC combination analgesics if previously successful

Choice of preventative medications
- Beta-adrenergic blocking agents
- Tricyclic antidepressants
- Anticonvulsants

Fig. 5.4 The US Primary Care Network Guidelines for migraine management.

booklet on patient-centred strategies for managing migraine in 2000. The Primary Care Network advocates the impact-based recognition of migraine and acute and preventative treatment strategies, together with special guidelines for using behavioural and physical treatments, treating chronic headache disorders and specific patient groups (*Fig. 5.4*).

Impact-based recognition of migraine involves the physician eliciting information on how headaches interfere with the patient's life, the frequency of headaches, any changes in headache pattern over the preceding 6 months and the previous use and effectiveness of headache medications (*see Q 8.4*). The guidelines for acute treatment are to abort migraine symptoms and disability within 2–4 hours of initiating therapy. Key tactics for achieving this are identified as providing patient education and instruction and tailoring intervention to the individual's needs. The Primary Care Network recommends treating migraine early in the attack when the headache is mild with triptans, NSAIDs, isometheptene or combination analgesics.

Migraine-specific treatments such as triptans are recommended if the headaches are likely to become moderate or severe. In practice, this includes most migraine patients, as nearly 85% of patients with significant impact associated with their migraines have attacks that routinely become moderate to severe. This follows recent clinical trial evidence that early intervention with triptans when the migraine headache is mild is the most effective treatment option for migraine. Preventative treatment is designed to reduce attack frequency, duration, severity and disability and prevent the development of chronic daily headache in patients with frequent headaches. Again, this involves patient education and instruction, plus the development of a formal management plan.

5.15 What practical general guidelines can be recommended for the primary care physician?

These three sets of guidelines have several recommendations in common:

- Patient counselling should be provided and their buy-in sought
- A careful diagnosis should be conducted
- Assessments of migraine impact should be used in the initial evaluation of patients
- An individual treatment plan should be produced for each patient – patients who have disabling migraine are recommended to have access to migraine-specific therapies from the outset
- Follow-up procedures should be implemented to monitor the outcome of therapy.

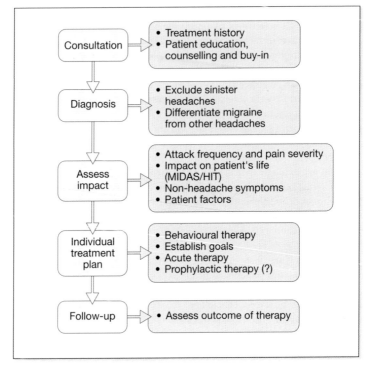

▲

Fig. 5.5 A proposed algorithm for individual patient management of migraine.

The rest of this section describes how these concepts can be translated into a practical scheme for the management of migraine and other headaches in primary care. Points 1–4 above need to be dealt with at the patient's initial consultation. Point 5 is dealt with at follow-up consultations. An algorithm for the management of migraine at the individual patient level is shown in *Figure 5.5*. These general principles also have application beyond migraine to all areas of headache management.

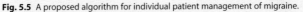

A PRACTICAL SCHEME FOR MIGRAINE MANAGEMENT IN PRIMARY CARE

5.16 How should headache consultations be arranged?

Headache is an important clinical condition and needs to be taken seriously by the patient and physician. To this end, a special consultation should be arranged when the typical situation occurs of a patient complaining of headache during a visit for another condition. In this way, the physician has sufficient time to evaluate the patient efficiently, while the patient realises that the physician takes their headache seriously and has time to prepare to discuss it in detail.

THE FIRST CONSULTATION

5.17 How do patients make the decision to consult a physician for migraine?

Studies have shown that migraine sufferers who consult a physician tend to be women who are severely affected by their attacks. People who have migraine with aura are also more likely to consult than those with migraine without aura.

It is likely that these patients may have exhausted OTC therapies and are consulting their physician as a last resort. Alternatively, they may be worried that the aura is symptomatic of a sinister condition. In both cases, they have real medical needs that require immediate attention.

5.18 What do patients bring to the first consultation?

Most migraine patients who consult a physician have suffered from the condition for several years. They therefore bring with them a history that can be ascertained with careful questioning. Migraine patients are frequently well educated about their condition and have a clear idea of what they are suffering from. This knowledge can be used to aid diagnosis and treatment choices.

On the other hand, some patients are at the end of their tether following years of suffering and may have to be managed carefully by the physician.

5.19 What should be achieved during the first headache consultation, and why is it so important?

By the end of the first consultation, the physician should have diagnosed the headache condition and either instituted an appropriate treatment or referred the patient to a specialist if a sinister headache is suspected. The physician should supply the patient with clear knowledge of their headache and what they should do to improve it. Both the physician and the patient need to agree on a management plan and how it is implemented and monitored. This is a lot to achieve but it has to be done to ensure that the patient adheres to the agreed management plan and does not lapse from care.

5.20 How can patient counselling and buy-in be achieved?

With most patients having a history of self-treating with OTC medications (and not always successfully), the first consultation may be the only opportunity the primary care physician has to manage the migraine effectively. Patients need to be shown that they are being listened to –use the consultation to formulate a constructive management plan. This will demonstrate to them that they are being well managed and encourage them to return for follow-up care. It is wise to make a specific appointment to discuss the patient's headache and to involve other members of the primary healthcare team, e.g. nurses and receptionists, to make optimal use of the time available.

5.21 How should the patient's treatment history be conducted?

Taking a headache history is a key task of the first consultation. Patients will already have tried OTC medications that may distort symptoms classically used in recognition and diagnosis. Patients may have also consulted a physician unsuccessfully in the past and tried prescribed therapies. The physician needs to know the patient's previous experience of headache management. In most instances history is taken when a person is not experiencing severe headache and hence the provider is obtaining a composite picture of that person's headaches over time. Given the wide range of symptoms that can occur from one migraine attack to another and the distortion of the natural evolution of a migraine that occurs with self-treatment effort, it is often best to have a patient focus first on their most problematic headache presentation. No single symptom defines migraine and the physician can use the history to create a clinical profile representative of the headache pattern. Ideally, the history should cover:

- Headache: the impact, type, severity, location, duration, frequency, timing and family history
- Other symptoms: visual, sensory and gastrointestinal
- Influencing factors: diet, lifestyle, hormonal and environmental
- Current medication taken for headaches and other conditions.

An example of a headache history card is shown in *Figure 5.6*. The nurse can help the patient to complete this card before they meet the physician. Nurses will meet many patients with headache at well-person clinics, routine vaccinations, antenatal, baby and family planning clinics, and can be proactive in this area.

5.22 How can patients be educated about their migraine?

Patients with a history of unsuccessful treatment may be sceptical of further medical care. They need to be shown that their physician takes migraine seriously and that new and effective therapies are available. People with headache are often motivated to understand their condition and physicians should provide them with information on the nature and mechanisms of

Headache History Card
Please tick the relevant box

Severity

___ Mild

___ Severe

Frequency

___ Several times a year

___ Several times a month

___ Several times a week

___ Once a year

___ Once a month

___ Once a week

Advance warning

___ Always

___ Sometimes

___ Never

What sort of warning do you get?

___ Visual disturbance

___ Numbness/tingling

___ Speech difficulties

___ Sensitivity to light

___ Feelings of weakness

___ None of the above

Where is the pain usually located?

___ Top of the head

___ Back of the head

___ One side of the head

___ Both sides of the head

___ Front of head

___ Other

How would you describe the pain?

___ An aching pain

___ A throbbing pain

___ A stabbing pain

___ A burning pain

___ None of these

Do you have any other symptoms during the headache?

___ Nausea/vomiting

___ Visual disturbance

___ Feelings of weakness

___ Speech difficulties

___ Loss of appetite

___ Dizziness

___ Sensitivity to light/noise

___ Numbness/tingling

Is the headache so bad you have to go to bed?

___ Always

___ Sometimes

___ Never

How long does your headache last?

___ Less than one hour

___ One to four hours

___ Four to six hours

___ Six to 12 hours

___ 12 to 24 hours

___ More than 24 hours

▲

Fig. 5.6 Example of a headache history card.

their disorder. The physician should have a range of leaflets available and can guide patients to the many professional organisations that can provide further information via publications or websites (see Appendix 2). The UK Migraine Action Association has a particularly useful booklet on migraine that is specifically designed for patient use (see references). There are also excellent short books on migraine and other headaches that the patient can purchase cheaply from pharmacists or bookshops (see references).

Patients should be told that even though primary headaches can not be cured the pain and other symptoms can be controlled and their impact minimised. An explicit understanding of realistic treatment goals can improve patient satisfaction with care.

5.23 How can patients self-manage their migraine?

As with other chronic conditions, patients need to manage their migraine themselves, making decisions about lifestyle alterations and how and when to take their medications. Physicians should encourage their patients to participate in their own management and effective communication between the physician and patient has been shown to improve care delivery. Patient preference is an important consideration in the choice of treatment. Patients may rate such factors as speed of response, overall headache relief, a lack of side effects or convenience as the most important characteristics of treatment.

5.24 How can the physician diagnose migraine with confidence and accuracy?

The first step in the effective management of headache is to make the correct diagnosis when the patient first consults. It is important that the patient is made to appreciate that they have a recognised disorder that is not trivial and which the primary care physician appreciates is distressing. Fortunately, recent diagnostic advances mean that the physician has clear guidelines for the differential diagnosis of migraine and other headaches.

Although serious secondary (sinister) headaches are rare, it must be stressed that an accurate diagnosis is essential to facilitate the successful management of migraine and other headaches in primary care. Headache diagnosis is covered in Section 3 and the physician is referred there for the necessary information. Using these criteria, diagnosis of migraine should be rapid and accurate. Additionally, it is often worth asking the patient what self-diagnosis they would give.

5.25 How can the severity of a patient's migraine be measured?

The physician needs to assess the patient's illness severity in order to select an appropriate medication. However, this is not as easy as it sounds. While pain intensity is the most important aspect of migraine to the individual sufferer and most patients consulting their physicians do so for pain relief, economic studies have shown that headache-related disability is the most important determinant of migraine's societal impact in economic terms. The new guidelines for migraine care recommend that the physician assesses the following criteria to determine illness severity:

- Attack frequency and pain severity
- The impact (disability) on the patient's life
- Associated nonheadache symptoms
- Patient factors, such as their response to prior medications, their preferences and their concurrent illnesses.

5.26 How can the impact of migraine on the patient's lifestyle be assessed?

Assessments of migraine impact have proved to be accurate measures of headache illness severity and two tools have been developed to assess this: the Migraine Disability Assessment (MIDAS) questionnaire and the Headache Impact Test (HIT).

5.27 What is the Migraine Disability Assessment (MIDAS) Questionnaire?

MIDAS is a paper-based questionnaire, designed to be accessible at physicians' surgeries and pharmacies. Migraine sufferers answer five disability questions in three activity domains covering the previous 3-month period (*Fig. 5.7*). They score the number of lost days due to headache in employment, household work and family and social activities. Sufferers also report the number of additional days with significant limitations to activity (defined as at least 50% reduced productivity) in the employment and household work domains. The total MIDAS score is obtained by summing the answers to the five questions as lost days due to headache. This can sometimes be higher than the actual number of lost headache days due to any one day being counted in more than one domain. The score is categorised into four severity grades:

- Grade I = 0–5 (defined as minimal or infrequent disability)
- Grade II = 6–10 (mild or infrequent disability)
- Grade III = 11–20 (moderate disability)
- Grade IV = 21 and over (severe disability).

Two other questions (A and B) are not scored, but are designed to provide the physician with clinically relevant information on headache frequency

This form can help you and your doctor improve the management of your headaches

Do You Suffer From

headaches?

MIDAS QUESTIONNAIRE

INSTRUCTIONS: Please answer the following questions about ALL your headaches you have had over the last 3 months. Write your answer in the box next to each question. Write zero if you did not do the activity in the last 3 months.

1 On how many days in the last 3 months did you miss work or school because of your headaches? ☐ days

2 How many days in the last 3 months was your productivity at work or school reduced by half or more because of your headaches? *(Do not include days you counted in question 1 where you missed work or school)* ☐ days

3 On how many days in the last 3 months did you not do household work because of your headaches? ☐ days

4 How many days in the last 3 months was your productivity in household work reduced by half or more because of your headaches? *(Do not include days you counted in question 3 where you did not do household work)* ☐ days

5 On how many days in the last 3 months did you miss family, social or leisure activities because of your headaches? ☐ days

TOTAL ☐ days

A On how many days in the last 3 months did you have a headache? *(If a headache lasted more than 1 day, count each day)* ☐ days

B On a scale of 0–10, on average how painful were these headaches? *(Where 0 = no pain at all, and 10 = pain as bad as it can be)* ☐

© Innovative Medical Research 1997

Once you have filled in the questionnaire, add up the total number of days from questions 1–5 (ignore A and B).

Grading system for the MIDAS Questionnaire:		
Grade	Definition	Score
I	Little or no disability	0–5
II	Mild disability	6–10
III	Moderate disability	11–20
IV	Severe disability	21+

MIDAS·

MIDAS is supported by an unrestricted educational grant from

AstraZeneca

▲

Fig. 5.7 The Migraine Disability Assessment (MIDAS) Questionnaire. The MIDAS programme was developed by Innovative Medical Research Inc, with sponsorship and assistance from AstraZeneca.

and pain intensity. Information on MIDAS can be accessed on-line at
www.migraine-disability.net.

5.28 How can the MIDAS Questionnaire be used?

MIDAS has been tested extensively and shown to be reliable and valid, with
wide potential for clinical utility. It can be used to:

- Improve communication between patients and their physicians on the
  impact of migraine
- Help the physician to assess illness severity
- Help the physician to produce an individualised treatment plan for
  each patient, when used with other clinical assessments
- Provide an outcome measure to monitor the success of interventions.

5.29 What is the Headache Impact Test (HIT)?

HIT was first developed as a web-based test, designed to be accessible to all
physicians and headache sufferers through the internet (at
www.headachetest.com and www.amIhealthy.com).

This is a dynamic questionnaire, with items derived from four validated
headache questionnaires sampling all areas of headache impact. Patients
are questioned until clinical standards of score precision are met. In
practice, five questions are sufficient to grade the majority of headache
sufferers with severe, moderate or mild headache. Internet-HIT
differentiates sufferers on the basis of diagnosis and characteristics such as
headache severity and frequency. The test takes only 1–2 minutes to complete.

HIT-6 is a paper-based, short-form questionnaire based on the Internet-
HIT question pool, designed for people without access to the internet
(*Fig. 5.8*). Six questions cover pain severity, loss of work and recreational
activities, tiredness, mood alterations and cognition. Each question is scored
on a five-point scale with the scores being added to produce the final score.
HIT-6 scores are categorised into four grades, representing minimal, mild,
moderate and severe impact due to headache. Internet-HIT and HIT-6
scores compared well to each other when the two forms of the
questionnaire were tested on a group of headache sufferers.

5.30 How can HIT be used?

Like MIDAS, HIT has been tested extensively and shown to be reliable and
valid, with wide potential for clinical utility. It can be used to:

- Improve communication between patients and their physicians on the
  impact of migraine

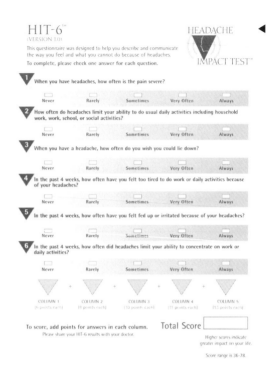

Fig. 5.8 The HIT-6 Questionnaire. HIT was developed by Quality Metric Inc and GlaxoSmithKline.

- Help the physician to diagnose migraine
- Help the physician to assess illness severity
- Help the physician to produce an individualised treatment plan for each patient, when used with other clinical assessments.

However, unlike MIDAS, it has not to date been tested as an outcome measure to monitor the success of interventions.

5.31 How can impact testing be best used in primary care?

Both MIDAS and HIT were developed to assess the whole spectrum of headache and are not restricted to migraine only. They are widely used by specialist physicians but so far have had limited uptake in primary care. Primary care physicians should be encouraged to use these tools to evaluate their patients. Patients should be encouraged to complete the forms before they see the physician, with help if needed from the receptionist or nurse at the surgery.

In addition to using the MIDAS or HIT assessment tool, it is often valuable to ask the patient to explain their expectations of headache management. Occasionally, patients may have infrequent high-impact migraines. In these cases the impact measures will not necessarily measure the true impact of the migraine to the individual patient and thus sole reliance on these measures is not recommended.

PROVIDING AN INDIVIDUALISED TREATMENT PLAN FOR EACH PATIENT

5.32 What are the principles underlying individualised management of migraine?

Owing to its inherent heterogeneity, migraine management needs to be tailored to each patient's individual needs. The following factors should be taken into consideration:

- Headache frequency
- Headache duration and severity
- Presence and severity of nonheadache associated symptoms
- Impact of headache on the patient's life, assessed with MIDAS or HIT
- The patient's history and preference.

5.33 How can the physician establish realistic goals with the patient?

It is important that physicians and patients share an understanding of the presenting headache and expectations of treatment. Patients may not fully understand their illness and/or may have expectations of treatment that are too high or too low. Physicians often do not define for themselves realistic expectations of interventions for migraine and instead rely on broad and often vague criteria for success.

For acute therapy, the IHS has suggested for research that the target should be that patients are pain-free 2 hours after intervention. While this stringent criterion may not be possible for every patient or with every migraine, it does set the ultimate standard by which patients and physicians can judge the success of treatment. More realistic targets for acute treatments may be to aim for:

- The patient to have mild or no headache at 2 hours after treatment, irrespective of the pretreatment severity
- The patient to express preference and/or satisfaction with the medication
- The patient to be able to resume their normal activities within 2 hours of treatment.

This latter target is perhaps of most relevance to the patient, bearing in mind the subjective nature of the perception of headache severity.

In order to avoid the complications of excessive analgesic overuse, it is valuable to set limits on the quantity of acute medications being consumed.

Many physicians have advocated that acute medications be taken < 2 days per week.

The primary goal of prophylactic therapy should be to reduce headache frequency by > 50% and/or improve a concurrent condition. Due to the risk of side effects with these therapies, they also need to be well tolerated. The patient should also express a preference and/or satisfaction with these therapies.

Once the physician and patient understand the presenting problem and the goals of therapy they can work together to expedite a formal management plan.

5.34 How can the patient's preferences be dealt with?

By working in partnership with the patient, the physician can ensure that patient preferences are incorporated into management plans and unrealistic fears and expectations overcome.

The physician should ensure that the patient's preferences are taken account of in treatment decisions for headache, provided they are realistic. Patients usually have a clear idea of those therapies that have proved useful in the past and those that have not worked. This can save valuable time in the selection of an initial medication that is likely to succeed.

Patients may prefer to use an acute or a prophylactic medication as first-line treatment – these preferences should be respected as far as possible. However, patients may also have illogical fears of certain medications that need to be overcome by the physician so that effective treatment can be provided.

5.35 How should behavioural and lifestyle therapies be provided?

Behavioural preventative strategies should be provided for every patient. This can include relaxation training and/or biofeedback and advice on trigger avoidance. About 20% of patients can reduce the frequency of their migraine attacks by identifying specific migraine triggers and avoiding them. However, all patients should be advised to take measures that could reduce the influence of migraine triggers:

- Eat and sleep regularly
- Try to manage stress and find ways to relax
- Try to avoid encountering several triggers simultaneously (e.g. don't drink red wine when under stress).

Behavioural and lifestyle therapies should be used in concert with effective acute and prophylactic medications as there is evidence that their effects may be synergistic.

Alternative therapies should not be discouraged as the patient may be convinced that they are of benefit. However, the physician should be aware of the potential side effects and interactions with conventional treatments that may occur.

5.36 How should decisions based on headache frequency be conducted?

The physician can assess headache frequency easily from the patient history or from Question A on a completed MIDAS form.

■ Patients with more than three or four migraine attacks per month should be offered prophylactic medication plus acute medication for breakthrough attacks
  ■ The prophylactic medications of choice are beta-blockers, sodium valproate/divalproex sodium and amitriptyline.
  ■ Menstrual migraine is sometimes managed with oral contraceptives, given as short-term prophylaxis during the perimenstrual period.
■ The physician should suspect chronic daily headache or cluster headache if the patient has more than 15 days of 'migraine-like' headache per month. – these patients are probably best referred to a specialist for care.
■ However, the majority of patients experience infrequent attacks and require acute medication only.

5.37 How can impact test results be integrated with headache diaries and other assessments?

Impact testing is not designed to be used on its own to evaluate patients but as part of a programme of evaluation to determine the burden of migraine to the patient. Also, impact testing is a relatively new concept – most primary care physicians have no experience of these procedures and will be unwilling to use them as a single assessment of migraine severity. However, they do provide a clinically valid measure of the impact of the migraine on the sufferer's life. Headache diaries and physician questioning can provide data on migraine frequency, duration, symptomatology and severity. This information, used together with that provided from impact testing, can provide the physician with all the information needed to make clinical decisions.

5.38 How should migraine symptoms be evaluated?

Patients with migraine often experience considerable variability in their headache presentations. They often have a spectrum of headaches, some of which are high impact and others low impact. In addition, their treatment needs can vary considerably based on the dynamics of their daily life. With these modifying factors in mind, it is valuable to divide patients into two categories, based on their assessed illness severity:

■ Mild to moderate intensity, requiring nonspecific therapies
■ Moderate to severe intensity, requiring migraine-specific therapies.

5.39 Does the patient have mild to moderate or moderate to severe migraine?

Patients with mild to moderate migraine have the following characteristics:

■ Headaches that are almost always mild to moderate in intensity (mild headaches are not generally seen in clinical practice).
■ Nonheadache associated symptoms, if present, are not severe in intensity.
■ The impact of the headache on the patient's lifestyle is not significant:
　■ MIDAS Grade I or II (minimal or mild disability)
　■ HIT Grade 1 or 2 (minimal or mild impact).

Patients with mild to moderate migraine may experience satisfactory benefit with aspirin or other NSAIDs in high doses, analgesic-antiemetic combinations or isometheptene-paracetamol combinations. Additional prophylactic medications may be required for patients with frequent headaches.

Patients with moderate to severe migraine have the following characteristics:

■ Headaches that frequently develop to moderate or severe in intensity.
■ Significant nonheadache associated symptoms, which may be severe in intensity.
■ The impact of the headache on the patient's lifestyle is significant:
　■ MIDAS Grade III or IV (moderate or severe disability)
　■ HIT Grade 3 or 4 (moderate or severe impact).

Patients with moderate to severe migraine should be prescribed from the outset migraine-specific drugs that have proven clinical evidence of efficacy. The triptans have the best clinical profile of these drugs and can be recommended for most patients. Ergotamine can no longer be recommended due to the risk of habituation and development of chronic daily headache. However, DHE can be used as an alternative to triptans, particularly where a long-acting effect is required. Additional prophylactic medications may be required for patients with frequent headaches.

CHOOSING THE OPTIMAL ACUTE THERAPY

5.40 When should acute treatments be used?

Acute treatments should be prescribed to all migraine patients, either as monotherapy for infrequent attacks or in conjunction with prophylactic medications for frequent attacks.

5.41 When should simple and combination analgesics be used?

Patients with mild to moderate migraine can be prescribed analgesics or combination therapies that have proven clinical evidence of efficacy, including:

■ Aspirin and NSAIDs, used in high doses (e.g. aspirin 900 mg)
■ Analgesic-antiemetic combination medications, e.g. aspirin plus metoclopramide, paracetamol plus metoclopramide or paracetamol plus domperidone
■ Isometheptene and paracetamol combination medications.

For maximal effect, the physician should advise the patient to take these medications as early as possible during the attack. If patients have clear signs and symptoms of an impending attack, they should take the medications before the headache starts. If they do not get these signs they should treat the attack as soon as the headache starts, while it is still mild in intensity.

However, the physician should realise that most patients will have already tried simple analgesics before they consult their physician. The physician needs to elicit the patient's treatment history before prescribing acute medications. Those who have failed previously on simple analgesics and combination medications should be prescribed a migraine-specific medication from the outset.

5.42 When should a triptan be used?

Triptans are not a 'miracle cure' for migraine but do have the best evidence for efficacy of any migraine-specific drugs. Triptans can be prescribed from the outset as first-line therapy to all patients with moderate to severe migraine who do not have contraindications for their use. They should also be used for patients who have failed on simple and combination analgesics.

5.43 Which patients should not be given triptans?

In general, triptans are contraindicated for patients with:
■ Evidence of existing cardiovascular disease
■ Uncontrolled hypertension
■ Severe renal and hepatic impairment.
The patient should be fully evaluated before receiving triptans if they:
■ Have risk factors for cardiovascular disease, e.g. history of smoking or men aged > 40 years

- Have controlled hypertension
- Have any renal or hepatic disease
- Show hypersensitivity reactions
- Are pregnant or breast-feeding.

These patients should only be prescribed triptans if the clinical benefits are likely to outweigh the associated risks of treatment.

Patients taking the following drugs generally should not be prescribed triptans: other triptans, ergotamine and its derivatives and MAOIs. Other drugs are proscribed for individual triptans and are considered later (*see Q 5.45*).

5.44 Which patients should receive oral triptans?

All the available oral triptans are effective and well tolerated acute treatments for migraine, but no one triptan is an unequivocal choice. However, some general principles for prescribing can be outlined:

- Most patients can be effectively treated with one of the oral triptans. Triptans are effective for migraine without aura and migraine with aura, and for migraine subtypes such as menstrual migraine and early morning migraine that is fully developed upon wakening.
- Sumatriptan, zolmitriptan, rizatriptan and almotriptan can be recommended as the best triptans for first-line use. Eletriptan is likely to have a similar clinical profile to these drugs but has not been available in clinical practice long enough to make an unequivocal decision.
- Naratriptan and frovatriptan can also be recommended for first-line use, although their efficacy may be lower than the other triptans.

Patients should be told to take their triptan at the start of the headache phase when the headache is mild. Until recently, patients were told to take their medication when the headache was established and moderate or severe in intensity. This advice followed the study design in triptan clinical trials. However, clinical evidence from the Spectrum study showed that sumatriptan was most effective when given early in the attack when the migraine headache was mild (*Fig. 5.9*). Recent evidence from studies with other oral triptans shows that they too are most effective when taken early in the attack.

Further evidence from the Spectrum study showed that sumatriptan was effective for the range of headaches experienced by migraine sufferers, including tension-type headache as well as migraine attacks. This indicates that triptans can be used to treat all headaches experienced by migraine sufferers, which simplifies their everyday use.

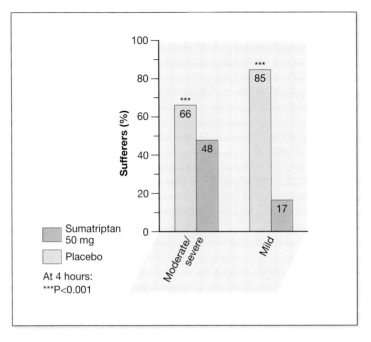

Fig. 5.9 Efficacy of sumatriptan 50 mg at 4 hours after treatment when given for mild or moderate/severe migraine headache.

5.45 Do all the oral triptans provide a similar level of efficacy and safety?

All the oral triptans are effective and well tolerated acute treatments for migraine. Despite the best efforts of the individual manufacturers to persuade otherwise, differences in their respective clinical profiles are small as elucidated from clinical studies and have not been demonstrated to date in clinical practice.

In an attempt to provide a personal perspective on the different oral triptans, the following information might be relevant:

■ Sumatriptan has now been available for over a decade in most countries and has a good clinical profile established in clinical practice. It is now the gold standard for other oral triptans to be compared to.

■ Naratriptan is not as effective as sumatriptan over the 2–4 hours after treatment but may be slightly better tolerated and is associated with less headache recurrence. However, it should not be co-administered with methysergide.

■ Zolmitriptan has a very similar clinical profile to sumatriptan, despite its greater lipophilicity and central penetrability. However, it should not be co-administered with cimetidine, fluvoxamine and quinolones.

■ Rizatriptan seems to have a slightly faster onset of action than sumatriptan and zolmitriptan, although the overall response rates of the three drugs are similar. However, it should not be co-administered with propranolol and drugs acting as cytochrome P450 CYP2D6 substrates.

■ Almotriptan has a similar efficacy profile to sumatriptan but may be slightly better tolerated and be associated with less headache recurrence. However, it should not be co-administered with lithium.

■ Eletriptan 80 mg seems to have a slightly faster onset of action than sumatriptan and zolmitriptan, while the 40 mg and 20 mg doses have clinical profiles similar to sumatriptan. However, safety problems may limit the use of eletriptan at the higher doses. It should not be co-administered with potent CYP3A4 inhibitors such as ketoconazole, itraconazole, erythromycin, clarithromycin, josamycin, and protease inhibitors such as ritonavir, indinavir and nelfinavir. There is also the possibility of abnormal liver function with the 80 mg dose.

■ Frovatriptan is not as effective as sumatriptan over the 2–4 hours after treatment but may be slightly better tolerated.

5.46 Is it sensible to switch between the oral triptans?

If a patient is effectively managed with an established oral triptan, there is no need to introduce a new triptan because of small theoretical improvements in efficacy that may be promoted by the manufacturers.

However, if one triptan is not effective, clinical study evidence indicates that an alternative triptan is likely to be effective and should be prescribed. There is anecdotal evidence of some patients becoming tolerant to one triptan, following months or years of effective treatment. In this case, switching to another triptan is usually effective.

5.47 Are the ODT triptan formulations preferable to the conventional oral tablet formulations?

The orally-disintegrating tablet (ODT) formulations of zolmitriptan and rizatriptan exhibit similar clinical profiles to the conventional tablet formulations. However, they are popular with patients and many patients prefer them.

If a patient has unpredictable migraine attacks or has difficulty in swallowing tablets during their attacks, it may be best to give them one of the ODT formulations of zolmitriptan or rizatriptan that can be taken at any time without water.

5.48 Which patients should receive nasal spray triptans?

The majority of migraine patients can be successfully managed with an oral triptan and these are considerably cheaper than the nasal spray and subcutaneous injection formulations.

However, patients who have rapidly-developing severe attacks may require a particularly fast-acting triptan. In this case, nasal spray sumatriptan or zolmitriptan may be an appropriate treatment. As yet there is no clinical evidence to distinguish between these two nasal spray formulations.

5.49 Which patients should receive subcutaneous sumatriptan?

Patients who have rapidly-developing severe attacks may require a particularly fast-acting triptan. In this case, subcutaneous sumatriptan may be appropriate. Patients with severe nausea or vomiting may be unable to take oral or nasal spray triptans – subcutaneous sumatriptan should be tried.

5.50 Are any triptans 'safer' to use than others?

All triptans are generally well tolerated with a characteristic profile of adverse events that are transient and mild to moderate in intensity. However, some patients do have difficulties in tolerating the symptoms of heaviness, pressure and pain that may accompany use of oral triptans. These patients can be given naratriptan or almotriptan, which seem to have fewer associated side effects than the other triptans.

5.51 Are any triptans effective in treating headache recurrence?

There has been much discussion among headache experts concerning the nature of headache recurrence and whether it represents a true return of the migraine or the development of another type of headache. Nevertheless, clinical studies of the triptans show that a second dose, taken when the headache returns within 2–24 hours of the first dose, can effectively treat recurrent headache.

Patients who experience frequent headache recurrence may benefit from the long-acting naratriptan or almotriptan, which have the least associated recurrence of any of the triptans. Other long-acting drugs, such as DHE, may also be useful for these patients.

5.52 Are any triptans effective as rescue medication?

A self-administered rescue medication should always be supplied to the patient to treat for nonresponse or headache recurrence. This is usually a second dose of the original triptan but some opiate analgesics may be provided in supervised conditions.

Subcutaneous sumatriptan is also a very useful rescue medication if oral and nasal spray formulations fail. Quite a few patients carry multiple sumatriptan formulations and reserve subcutaneous sumatriptan for rescue or for the treatment of particularly severe attacks. This can be a very effective use of the stratified/staged care treatment strategy (*see Q 4.8*).

5.53 Is there a place for ergotamine and DHE in migraine management?

Ergotamine is no longer recommended as an acute treatment for migraine – a European consensus meeting concluding that triptans were generally a better option. The only time to use ergotamine is with patients experienced with its use and dosage restrictions, who do not want to switch to triptans, and who experience infrequent or long-duration attacks. The rectal route should be used for these patients, although ergotamine suppositories are not available in all countries (including the UK).

Injection and nasal spray formulations of DHE are markedly inferior to equivalent triptan formulations and should not generally be used as first-line acute therapies for migraine. However, they may be useful for patients with long duration headaches or in those who experience regular headache recurrence with the triptans (*DHE is not currently available in the UK*).

5.54 Is there a place for opiate analgesics and barbiturates in migraine management?

In general, codeine and other opiates should not be used for the acute treatment of migraine, due to the risk of dependence and chronic daily headache. The physician should ask the patient if they take codeine-containing drugs for their migraine and, if so, provide them with alternative medications.

Opiate analgesics, including codeine, parenteral opiates and butorphanol (*not available in the UK and Europe*) may be used as emergency care for migraine that is resistant to treatment. These drugs should be provided in a supervised environment and records kept so that patients do not become habituated.

5.55 Can acute treatment be provided for each phase of the migraine attack?

Phase-specific treatment of migraine is a new concept currently under review and is discussed further in Section 8 (*see Q 8.5*). However, certain therapies are suited to be given during different phases of the migraine attack and, in terms of what the primary care practitioner can supply:

- Stress reduction, biofeedback, relaxation, naratriptan, DHE, aspirin, NSAIDs and combination analgesics may all be useful if taken during the prodrome and aura phases before the headache develops
- Triptans should optimally be taken early in the headache phase, when it is mild
- Triptans can also be taken later in the headache phase, when it is moderate to severe in intensity
- Triptans, opiates and parenteral antiemetics may all be taken as rescue therapy
- Simple analgesics, NSAIDs and rehydration therapy may all be useful in the recovery phase.

CHOOSING THE OPTIMAL PROPHYLACTIC THERAPY

5.56 When should prophylaxis be used?

Migraine prophylaxis is usually prescribed in the following situations:

- The patient suffers from more than 3–4 attacks per month
- Acute treatment is ineffective
- The patient has concurrent illnesses that mean effective acute therapies cannot be used
- The patient is at risk of over-using acute medications and therefore developing chronic daily headache
- The patient has one of the rare migraine subtypes, such as hemiplegic or basilar migraine, migraine with prolonged aura or migrainous infarction.

5.57 Can triptans ever be used as preventative treatments?

In general, triptans are used as acute medications only. Their short half-lives and duration of action make them unsuitable for chronic use, as they would have to be taken several times per day. Subcutaneous and oral triptans failed to prevent the migraine headache from developing when given during the aura phase.

However, the longer-acting triptans, such as naratriptan and frovatriptan, may have the potential to be used for prophylaxis in certain circumstances. Small studies have shown that naratriptan shows promise for the prophylaxis of transformed migraine and cluster headache, the short-term prophylaxis of menstrually-associated migraine during the perimenstual period and the prevention of migraine during the prodrome phase of the attack. No such studies have been conducted to date with frovatriptan. While naratriptan, and possibly frovatriptan, show promise in these areas, further studies are required to confirm these clinical effects before these drugs can be generally recommended for prophylaxis.

5.58 Which patients should receive beta-blockers?

Beta-blockers are effective and generally well tolerated prophylactic treatments for migraine. Most patients requiring prophylaxis are likely to start treatment with a beta-blocker, usually propranolol – although timolol, atenolol, metoprolol and nadolol may also be used.

Beta-blockers are particularly useful for patients with concurrent hypertension or angina, where they also have a clinical effect. However, they are contraindicated for patients with concurrent asthma, depression, congestive heart failure, Raynaud's disease and diabetes.

5.59 Which patients should receive sodium valproate / divalproex sodium?

Valproate is an effective and generally well tolerated prophylactic drug for migraine, and can be used for first-line therapy. It is especially useful if the patient has concurrent epilepsy, mania, anxiety disorders or chronic daily headache, where it also has a clinical effect. However, it is contraindicated for patients with liver disease, bleeding disorders and women who are planning to become pregnant.

5.60 Which patients should receive tricyclic antidepressants?

The tricyclic antidepressant amitriptyline is an effective and reasonably well tolerated prophylactic drug for migraine and can be used for first-line therapy. It is especially useful if the patient has concurrent depression, anxiety, insomnia or chronic daily headache, where it also has a clinical effect. However, it is contraindicated for patients with heart block, mania and urinary retention, and is sedating.

5.61 Which patients should receive calcium channel antagonists?

Calcium channel antagonists are moderately effective for migraine prophylaxis but are associated with a lot of side effects. They are also not generally available in many countries, including the UK and the USA. Where available, calcium channel antagonists are probably best restricted to second-line therapy. They may be especially useful if the patient has migraine with aura, and concurrent hypertension, angina or asthma, where they also have clinical effects. However, they are contraindicated for patients with constipation and hypotension.

5.62 Is there a place for 5-HT$_2$ antagonists as migraine prophylaxis?

5-HT$_2$ antagonists are moderately effective for migraine prophylaxis but are associated with a lot of side effects. They are therefore probably best restricted to second-line therapy. They may be useful if the patient has orthostatic hypotension, where they also have clinical effects, but are contraindicated for patients with angina and peripheral vascular disease. Due to its 5-HT$_1$ receptor activity, methysergide should probably not be co-administered with triptans and ergots. 5-HT$_2$ antagonists also tend to cause a significant amount of weight gain, which makes them unpopular amongst the young and middle-aged women who form such a large proportion of migraine sufferers.

5.63 Is there a place for DHE and NSAIDs as migraine prophylaxis?

There is little evidence for the use of DHE and NSAIDs for migraine prophylaxis and they should generally be avoided. Long-term use can lead to leg ischaemia and ergotism with DHE, gastrointestinal irritation with NSAIDs and chronic daily headache with both drugs.

5.64 Is there a place for alternative treatments in migraine prophylaxis?

Several alternative prophylactic therapies, such as feverfew, acupuncture, riboflavin and magnesium, all show some efficacy in migraine prevention. The physician can recommend all these therapies if the patient shows interest and wants to try something new. However, effective acute medications should always be available, as these therapies are no more a 'cure' than any of the conventional prophylactic agents.

FOLLOW-UP CONSULTATIONS

5.65 How can follow-up consultations be set up at the initial consultation?

Once the first consultation is over, it is important to set in place follow-up procedures to motivate patients to persevere with their treatment and return to the clinic for further care. A good way to do this is to issue a headache/migraine diary (*Fig. 5.10*), asking the patient to return in a few weeks with the completed diary. A MIDAS or HIT Questionnaire can also be given out at this time. The practice nurse can issue these forms and provide guidance if necessary.

5.66 How can the outcome of initial therapy be assessed and follow-up strategies implemented?

At follow-up assessments, the physician can use the completed diary cards and HIT score to confirm the diagnosis and the diary cards and MIDAS Questionnaire to objectively assess the efficacy of treatment. The MIDAS score typically decreases following successful treatment. For instance, patients may improve from a MIDAS Grade IV (score = 21+) to a Grade II (score = 5–10). Follow-up treatment decisions can then be made:

Managing migraine								

Severity of your symptoms

Please put a ✔(yes) or ✗(no) in the appropriate box Record whether you had the following symptoms	Date of attack ..../..../....		Date of attack ..../..../....		Date of attack ..../..../....		Date of attack ..../..../....	
	✔	or ✗	✔	or ✗	✔	or ✗	✔	or ✗
Headache								
Feeling sick								
Vomiting								
Other symptoms, e.g. sensitivity to light, sensitivity to noise, visual disturbances, speech difficulties, numbness (list these on the back page)								

The last treatment you tried

Write down the last treatment you took for your headache/migraine				

The effectiveness of your treatment

Please put a ✔(yes) or ✗(no) in the appropriate box	✔	or ✗	✔	or ✗	✔	or ✗	✔	or ✗
Did the treatment get rid of your migraine/headache?								
Did the treatment stop you feeling sick?								
Did the treatment treat all of your other symptoms?								
Please tick (✔) the statement which applies to you After taking the treatment, did you have to do any of these?	✔					✔		✔
Lie in a darkened room								
Sleep								
Leave work								
Stop what you were doing								
How many tablets did you take for your migraine attacks?								
One								
More than one								
After taking this treatment, how long was it before you started to feel its effect?								
30 mins or less								
Over 30 mins but less than 1 hour								
1 hour or more								
It did not work								
Please put a ✔(yes) or ✗(no) in the appropriate box	✔	or ✗						✗
Did you experience any side-effects from your treatment?								
Was the treatment better than ones you have tried before?								
Please tick (✔) the statement which applies to you In terms of your level of satisfaction with this migraine medication would you say:	✔						✔	
I was satisfied								
I was dissatisfied and would like to try a different medication								
I would value the opportunity to discuss treatment choices with my doctor								

Managing migraine
Headache/Migraine Diary card

Your name:
Date of birth:
Address:

Postcode:

Please use this diary to record details of the next four headache/migraine attacks you suffer. It will provide you, your pharmacist and your doctor with useful information and help you to find the best possible treatment to deal with your headache/migraine

Write today's date here:

Agree a date to review your headache/migraine and write that date here:

Fig. 5.10 Example of a headache/migraine diary.

- Patients who were treated effectively should continue with that therapy
- Patients who have failed on analgesics or combination medications should be provided with migraine-specific medications, usually a triptan
- Patients who have failed on a triptan can be provided with an alternative triptan
- Patients who find their triptan effective but inconvenient to use can be provided with an alternative formulation that suits their needs better
- Patients refractory to triptans, or who require regular rescue therapy, may require opiate drugs such as butorphanol or codeine-containing drugs for rescue. However, due to the danger of habituation and chronic daily headache, it is probably best to refer these patients to a specialist for treatment.

5.67 How should prophylactic medications be managed at follow-up?

Prophylaxis is not intended as a long-term management strategy but should be reviewed after 3 months. If the treatment is effective, without causing chronic side effects, treatment can be continued up to 6 months. If not, an alternative prophylactic drug can be supplied. At 6 months, the prophylactic can be withdrawn if the frequency of attacks is reduced. Providing the frequency remains reduced after withdrawal, it may be appropriate to revert to acute treatments only.

Patients who are refractory to repeated acute and/or prophylactic medications may need to be referred to a specialist for further care.

MANAGEMENT OF MIGRAINE IN SPECIAL POPULATIONS

5.68 How should children with migraine be managed?

As children with migraine may present with different symptoms to those of adults (*see Q 1.11*), diagnosis is a key feature of management (*see Q 3.10*). Following diagnosis, treatment of children with migraine should be conservative:

- If trigger factors are present, strategies for their minimisation should be implemented. This usually involves implementation of a regular lifestyle and meals.
- Paracetamol (with or without added antiemetics) is probably the first-line acute treatment. Aspirin can be introduced once the child is over 12 years of age. The role of triptans is controversial. While the oral triptans are effective, they tend to be no better than placebo and probably should be avoided. If a triptan is required, nasal spray sumatriptan or zolmitriptan is probably the best option.

■ Prophylactic therapies should be avoided if at all possible, as they are all associated with significant side effects.

5.69 How should men with migraine be managed?

Men with migraine can be problematic, as they tend not to consult their physicians for medical care. This may mean that when they do go to see their physician the symptoms and their impact may be severe. However, diagnosis and treatment of migraine in men should be straightforward. It should be borne in mind that what a man describes as migraine may well be cluster headache – careful differential diagnosis is therefore needed.

The prescription of triptans needs to be monitored in men, particularly those with cardiovascular risk factors, e.g. aged over 40 years, a history of smoking and family history of hypertension or cardiovascular disease. Patients who develop significant cardiovascular risk factors may need to be withdrawn from triptan therapy.

5.70 How should women of child-bearing age with migraine be managed?

Adolescent and young women are the most common group of patients with migraine seen in the physician's surgery. Diagnosis and management of this population is generally conventional and should pose no problems, as the incidence of other risk factors is low.

MENSTRUAL MIGRAINE

Many women report migraine attacks associated with their menstrual periods but usually have attacks at other times during the menstrual cycle. About 10% of women report only menstrual migraine attacks. Menstrually and nonmenstrually associated migraine attacks can both be managed with conventional acute and prophylactic therapies. Oestrogen supplements or NSAIDs are sometimes prescribed for short-term prophylaxis during the perimenstrual period but these are not always effective and should probably be reserved for patients in whom conventional therapies are ineffective. Avoiding migraine trigger factors and treating premenstrual symptoms with vitamin B6 or evening primrose oil may be a useful adjunct to prescription drugs.

ORAL CONTRACEPTION

Most women taking the contraceptive pill do not report any change in their migraine attacks. However, migraine may improve on starting the pill or the pattern of attacks may change, shifting to severe attacks during the pill-free week at the time of the period. It is generally safe for women with migraine to continue taking the pill, although women experiencing migraine with aura who have cardiovascular risk factors should take a low-oestrogen pill due to the very low risk of migrainous infarction (*see Q 2.10*). If women who normally have migraine without aura experience aura symptoms after starting the pill, the pill should be withdrawn and another form of contraception used. Women using the contraceptive pill can generally use the available acute and prophylactic medications, unless they have other concomitant risk factors.

5.71 How should pregnant and breast-feeding women with migraine be managed?

Migraine often improves during pregnancy, especially in the second and third trimesters, even though it may initially worsen during the first trimester. The migraine usually resumes its previous pattern post partum. This is conventionally explained by the high and stable oestrogen levels during pregnancy which decrease rapidly thereafter. However, this does not explain the story fully, as some migraine sufferers experience no change to their pattern of attacks during pregnancy and, in rare cases, migraine may appear for the first time during pregnancy.

Treatment of migraine is severely constrained during pregnancy. However, behavioural and stress reduction strategies can be maintained unchanged. Acute therapy is generally restricted to large doses of paracetamol (1000 mg), although aspirin and other NSAIDs can be taken during the first and second trimesters. Triptans and ergots are all contraindicated for pregnant and breast-feeding women. Prophylactic therapy is rarely indicated and only the beta-blockers may be used.

5.72 How should women with migraine taking hormone replacement therapy (HRT) be managed?

Little is known about the effects of taking HRT on the pattern of migraine attacks. Patients may experience more, or fewer, migraine attacks after starting to take HRT. The only way for the physician to find out is for the individual patient to try it and keep a headache diary. If the HRT used leads to an increased incidence of migraine attacks after an adequate trial, the type of HRT or route of administration can be changed. In general, patients' acute and prophylactic migraine therapies do not need to be changed when they start using HRT.

5.73 How should old people with migraine be managed?

Migraine usually decreases in prevalence as people move into old age but may persist. Some patients experience migraine throughout their lives. However, other headaches that can mimic migraine may also develop in older people, such as trigeminal and postherpetic neuralgias and temporomandibular joint dysfunction. A careful diagnostic procedure must therefore be instigated for

TABLE 5.4 Relative indications and contraindications for the use of migraine prophylaxis drugs

Prophylactic therapy	Contraindicated for use in concurrent illnesses	Indicated for use in concurrent illnesses
Beta-blockers	Asthma, depression, congestive heart failure, Raynaud's disease, diabetes	Hypertension, angina
Anticonvulsants: Sodium valproate/divalproex sodium	Liver disease, bleeding disorders	Epilepsy, mania, anxiety disorders, chronic headache disorders
Antidepressants: Amitriptyline	Mania, urinary retention, heart block	Depression, other headache and pain disorders, anxiety disorders, insomnia
Serotonin antagonists	Angina, peripheral vascular disease, glaucoma, renal impairment	Orthostatic hypertension, anorexia
Calcium channel antagonists	Hypotension, constipation	Hypertension, angina, asthma, migraine with aura

these patients, particularly in those who present with new onset headaches, to differentiate migraine from these, and sinister headaches.

Behavioural therapies should always be used with older people and some alternative strategies may also be useful. Many older people suffer from serious concurrent illnesses that require lifetime therapy, which can lead to a modification of antimigraine therapy. Triptans have been little studied in patients aged over 65 years and their use is generally discouraged in this age group. The older patient should be carefully evaluated for risk before a triptan is prescribed. In general, simple and combination analgesics have to be used as acute therapies. Prophylactic drugs may be contraindicated for patients with certain conditions but, on the other hand, may have the potential for synergistic action on other illnesses as well as migraine (*Table 5.4*).

5.74 How should different ethnic groups with migraine be managed?

Migraine is common in all ethnic groups, although it is more prevalent in white than in African or Asian races (*see Q 2.6*). This means that the physician will have migraine sufferers from all racial subgroups in their practice. The diagnosis and management of migraine does not differ in different races. However, careful questioning may be required for certain races where headache may not be considered a 'socially justifiable' illness.

5.75 How should people from different socioeconomic groups with migraine be managed?

Migraine affects all people in society more or less equally (*see Q 2.7*). Unfortunately, the physician may see fewer lower class than middle class migraine sufferers but this is probably due to the latter's greater tendency to consult a physician for medical care. The diagnosis and management of migraine does not differ in patients from different strata of society.

5.76 Do any patients with migraine require scanning procedures?

In general, very few headache sufferers require scanning procedures to confirm their diagnosis. People with the common benign headaches of migraine, tension-type headache and chronic daily headache can be diagnosed and treated effectively without the need for such procedures. Even patients with the rarer conditions of cluster headache and short, sharp headache can usually be managed in specialist care clinics without the need for scanning. The vast majority of scanning investigations are negative and are often conducted to reassure the patient that nothing is wrong. However, scanning procedures may be indicated where sinister headaches and the rare migraine subvariants are suspected.

PQ PATIENT QUESTIONS

5.77 Who should I see for my migraine?

Many migraine sufferers try to treat their attacks themselves, usually unsuccessfully. Most sufferers need help from a medical practitioner. The best source of advice and treatment is the primary care doctor, who can provide the most effective prescription treatments that are not available elsewhere. Pharmacists are also a useful source of advice and treatment, although they cannot provide the most effective medications. Some patients find it valuable to consult an alternative practitioner for care but these should not be used as the sole avenue of medical care.

5.78 How will the doctor deal with my migraine?

For the consultation with your doctor to work, you need to provide a clear history of your headache. It is worth thinking about this in advance and maybe writing down the key features of your headache. Your doctor will want to evaluate your headache history, diagnose your migraine, assess the severity of your illness and provide you with a treatment that will help you.

It is important that you work closely with your doctor during this process, letting them know your wishes and preferences. At the end of the consultation, you should have a clear plan for your treatment and a future appointment to check your progress.

5.79 Is there a cure for migraine?

There is no cure for migraine but it can be managed effectively in almost all cases. Successful people who have migraine are found in all walks of life. Migraine reflects the way the nervous system works and attacks occur when the nervous system is stimulated by an external source. Adjusting lifestyle, understanding how the nervous system works and certain drugs can help to prevent migraine attacks occurring. When they do occur, pain-killing and migraine-specific medications can stop them and allow the return of normal functioning.

5.80 What can be done to prevent migraine?

The basis for preventing migraine is to understand the causes of the attacks and, as far as possible, to minimise them. Learning to avoid or modify environmental and dietary factors likely to provoke migraine and creating positive coping and lifestyle strategies to reduce stress are all useful. Nonpharmacological strategies such as biofeedback and relaxation training can also prevent migraine. There is also a wide range of prophylactic drugs that can be used if needed. Alternative therapies such as acupuncture, herbs, vitamins and minerals, though not as thoroughly studied, may also be useful.

5.81 Do I need drugs every day to prevent migraine?

Most people with migraine do not need preventative medications. However, if migraines are frequent or difficult to treat, preventative medications can be invaluable. The purpose of preventative medications is to provide support to the nervous system so that it can effectively resist migraines. In most instances, many different factors put the nervous system at risk for migraine and consequently preventative medications need to be taken daily. Sometimes, when there is a predictable time or risk factor, such as a woman's period, a preventative medication may be taken only around that event. In most instances these medications only need to be used for a limited period of time. Lifestyle adjustments or establishing strategies to modify risk factors can be valuable additions to prescribed medications, and often limit the need for them.

Preventative medications may also be used if no acute treatment has proved effective or if the patient wishes to use therapies on a regular basis to prevent migraine.

5.82 What drugs will I need to treat my migraine attacks?

Almost all people use some kind of medication to treat their attacks of migraine when they occur (acute treatments) but the medication does not work very well for nearly half of them. The range of medications available varies considerably. Common medications include a variety of prescription and over-the-counter pain-killers, prescription medications for nausea, and specific prescription medications for migraine, which are the most effective therapies. Prescription medications may be in the form of tablets, nasal sprays or injections. Many patients use more than one type of medication or combinations of these products to treat their attacks. The most important features of a medication for treating migraine are that it safely and consistently stops the migraine and rapidly restores normal activities.

Management of nonmigraine headaches in primary care

6.1 What are the principles for managing nonmigraine headaches in primary care?

The basic principles of managing migraine in primary care are applicable to all headaches. The system of history taking, formal diagnosis, assessment of severity, prescription of appropriate therapy (or referral for specialist review) and follow-up should be followed in all cases. A clear differential diagnosis is the most important feature of managing the nonmigraine headaches, as this drives the choice of available management options.

6.2 How should the primary care physician manage the patient with suspected sinister headache?

Patients suspected of having sinister headaches following history taking and differential diagnosis procedures (*see* Qs 3.6, 3.27–33) require thorough evaluation. Usually this is accomplished by referral to a hospital or to a specialist, depending on the nature and seriousness of the condition.

6.3 How should the primary care physician manage the patient with tension-type headache?

Tension-type headache is the usual diagnosis for a dull, diffuse headache that does not impact significantly on the patient's lifestyle. It can occur in patients of all ages and can be episodic or chronic. In spite of it being the most common headache, episodic tension-type headache is seen relatively infrequently in primary care. Sufferers usually find over-the-counter (OTC) medications such as aspirin, paracetamol and nonsteroidal anti-inflammatory drugs (NSAIDs) effective and do not consult their physician for care. Physicians may see patients with chronic tension-type headaches and should treat them as having chronic daily headache (*see* Q 6.6).

Many patients with migraine also suffer from tension-type headaches. In these cases, the tension-type headache seems to arise via the same mechanisms as migraine and is part of the spectrum of headaches experienced by migraine sufferers (*see* Q 3.12). All headaches, including tension-type headache, experienced by migraine sufferers can be considered part of the migraine process and treated effectively with a triptan.

6.4 How should the primary care physician manage the patient with short sharp headaches?

Patients with short, sharp headaches are usually young adults who may think that they have migraine. However, short, sharp headaches are simple to diagnose due to their very short duration. Reassurance that the symptoms are benign is usually all that is required for patients with this type of headache. Patients who demand treatment may be best referred to a specialist. However, daily nonsteroidal NSAIDs can be provided. Indomethacin is the gold standard as it causes fewer gastrointestinal side effects than other NSAIDs (*see Q 4.125*).

6.5 How should the primary care physician manage the patient with cluster headache?

Many patients with cluster headache believe that they have migraine. However, it is relatively simple to diagnose due to the daily pattern of the headaches, their short duration and the predominance of the condition among young and middle-aged men (*see Q 3.17*).

After diagnosis, patients with cluster headache are best referred to a specialist for management. Subcutaneous sumatriptan 6 mg is the gold standard for abortive treatment. Oxygen inhalation may also be useful if the patient has access to the necessary high flow-rate equipment. Prophylaxis with prednisolone, methysergide or ergotamine (short-term), or verapamil or lithium (long-term) is also usually prescribed (*Table 6.1*) (*see Q 4.126*).

TABLE 6.1 Effective treatments for cluster headache	
Abortive treatments	**Prophylactic treatments**
Subcutaneous sumatriptan 6 mg	*Short-term*
Oxygen inhalation	Prednisolone (transitional only)
	Methysergide
	Ergotamine daily (nocturnal)
	Long-term
	Verapamil
	Lithium

6.6 How should the primary care physician manage the patient with chronic daily headache?

Chronic daily headaches are common in all age groups. Any headache that occurs for > 4 hours on > 15 days per month can be classified as chronic daily headache (*see Q 1.17*). However, this provides no information on the type of headache or its causes. Careful history and symptom taking is necessary to elicit this information. Most chronic daily headaches are of the following types:

- ■ Chronic tension-type headaches
- ■ Chronic migraines
- ■ Episodic migraines superimposed over a daily pattern of chronic tension-type headaches (the most frequently seen type).

Management of chronic daily headaches can be complex, depending on their aetiology, and such cases are probably best referred to a neurologist or headache specialist following diagnosis in primary care. The most frequent causes of chronic daily headache are abuse of analgesics and other headache medications and a history of head injury. Management involves avoidance of analgesics, physical measures to the neck, and appropriate prophylactic and acute treatments (*see Q 4.127*).

6.7 How should the primary care physician manage the patient with sinus headache?

Sinus headaches secondary to infectious aetiology can be experienced by all age groups. After diagnosis, the physician can provide a broad-spectrum antibiotic and recommend steam inhalation or vasoconstrictor agents for local treatment. Oral decongestants can be provided if treatment is required for more than 72 hours. If this fails, it is probably best to refer the patient to a specialist (*see Q 4.128*).

However, misdiagnosis is perhaps the greatest pitfall with sinus headache. A positive diagnosis of sinusitis is required. Evidence of acute sinusitis, with a purulent discharge from the nose, and support with imaging or using a flexible scope, can confirm the diagnosis (*see Qs 3.21, 3.22*). In the absence of this evidence, migraine may be a more likely diagnosis.

6.8 How should the primary care physician manage the patient with trigeminal neuralgia?

Trigeminal neuralgia is mostly found in older people, where it may present with migraine-like symptoms. However, the frequency, duration and character of the pain allows for a straightforward diagnosis (*see Q 3.23*). Following diagnosis, the physician should prescribe carbamazepine. If this or alternative drugs do not control the symptoms (*see Q 4.129*), referral for surgery may be appropriate.

6.9 How should the primary care physician manage the patient with postherpetic neuralgia?

Postherpetic neuralgia is usually found in older people and physicians treating patients with Herpes zoster should be aware of this complication. Diagnosis of the zoster may be complicated by the presence of mild or hidden lesions, however. Treatment for the neuralgia is dependent on the stage of the herpes infection, with one of three strategies being used:

- Antiviral drugs during the acute eruption of pain
- Analgesics and topical applications in the acute phase of the rash
- Tricyclic antidepressants and local application of capsaicin once the rash has cleared (*see Q 4.129*).

6.10 How should the primary care physician manage the patient with temporomandibular joint dysfunction?

Temporomandibular joint dysfunction is again mostly a condition of older people. Following a diagnosis of this condition (*see Q 3.26*), the best management option for the primary care physician is to refer the patient to a dentist for care. The physician can provide additional stress management programmes and prophylaxis with a tricyclic antidepressant.

6.11 How does the management of headache change during different life stages?

The diagnosis and management (*see Qs 5.68–73*) of headache change with the age of the presenting patient. In general, preteenage children, pregnant women and nursing mothers are managed conservatively with many medications contraindicated. The rule is that the benefits of treatment must outweigh any risk to the patient.

For teenagers and young to middle-aged men, and women taking adequate contraceptive measures, most medications are appropriate, provided other risk factors are not present. Older patients, however, often have serious concurrent illnesses that can limit the headache medications that can be prescribed. Each patient must be evaluated carefully.

PQ **PATIENT QUESTIONS**

6.12 What is the best way to treat my tension headaches?

Treatment for tension-type headache is best determined by the circumstances that accompany the headache:

- If tension-type headache is isolated and the only type of headache a person experiences, it can be self-treated with rest, sleep, exercise and a simple nonprescription painkiller. Usually it is not necessary to see a doctor for treatment.
- If tension-type headaches are frequent, then preventative medications are probably required and you should see your doctor for care.
- If tension headache is often associated with migraine attacks, they may well be part of the migraine process and can be treated as such. You should certainly see your doctor.
- If tension headache is a component of a pattern of daily headaches, then medical care is essential and you should go to see your doctor.

6.13 My husband gets excruciating headaches several times a day, but won't go to the doctor. What can I do?

From your description, your husband probably has a condition known as cluster headache. Sufferers, who are mostly men, experience short-lasting but very severe headaches several times a day for periods of weeks or months (or, less frequently, on a constant basis). Cluster headache is rare but can be treated and does not indicate a serious illness. However, prescription medications are needed for treatment and your husband must go to his doctor to receive this medical care.

6.14 I get headaches every day. What can I do?

Daily headaches are a problem for doctors and patients alike. Having daily headaches suggests that the nervous system itself is sensitised and its pain-suppressing abilities impaired. Many factors may be associated with the development of chronic daily headaches, including head injury and genetic factors. Probably the most important causative factor, because it is treatable, is the overuse of painkillers used to treat attacks of migraine. Whenever daily headaches are associated with daily use of headache medication, then that medication itself may be perpetuating the headache. Typical of this condition is a history of episodic headache in earlier life that over time evolves into a daily headache pattern. Once established, the offending medication may temporarily relieve the headache but as the medicine is excreted the headache returns, requiring more medication, which continues the cycle. Medicines that commonly cause daily headaches are codeine, ergotamine, barbiturates, and caffeine-containing products.

The key to managing daily headaches is to discontinue the use of the offending medication. This generally requires medical assistance and sometimes a short stay in hospital.

6.15 Antibiotics don't work for my sinus headaches. What can I do?

Many people commonly experience head and facial pain localised to the sinus area. Infrequently, this can be part of an infectious process called sinusitis. In these instances antibiotics are typically prescribed. However, far more often, recurrent episodes of pain in this area associated with nasal congestion or even tears in the eyes are migraine attacks. Ironically, migraine is a far more frequent cause of these symptoms than is a sinus infection. These symptoms occur during migraine because the same nerve that goes to blood vessels around the brain also goes into the sinus area. If branches of that nerve are activated during migraine then nasal symptoms are seen.

It is important that you receive an accurate diagnosis for your headache, and you should certainly go to see your doctor.

6.16 I have just had an attack of shingles and am getting awful headaches. What can I do?

You are probably suffering from a condition called postherpetic neuralgia. This often follows attacks of shingles and the pain can be very severe. It is important that you go back to your doctor for treatment, as this condition is unlikely to get better on its own for a long time.

7.1 What is a primary care headache team?

The management of headache in primary care is, of necessity, a long-term business. Patients need to be evaluated and treated carefully over a period of time. The physician's time and energy can be conserved during this process by using other members of the primary healthcare team.

The primary care headache team includes the physician, practice nurse and receptionists. Outside healthcare providers may also be involved, including community pharmacists, community nurses, opticians, dentists and providers of alternative medicine. Specialist physicians can be used for certain headaches and when treatment fails. Last, but not least, the patient must be an integral part of the team.

7.2 What is the role of the community pharmacist?

The community pharmacist is an integral part of the primary care headache team. The pharmacist is often the first source of healthcare advice that headache sufferers use and may well see them at the time of an attack. The pharmacist can:

- Educate headache sufferers about their condition
- Identify some migraine sufferers and provide them with over-the-counter (OTC) medications that may be effective
- Advise appropriate sufferers to consult their primary care physician
- Encourage sufferers to go back to their physician if their current prescribed medication is not working.

7.3 What is the role of the practice nurse?

The practice nurse can conduct much of the evaluation of the patient before they see the physician:

- Completing a headache history and Migraine Disability Assessment (MIDAS) or Headache Impact Test (HIT) evaluation
- Explaining about migraine and the medications used to treat it
- Giving out and evaluating headache diary cards
- Advocating the early use of OTC medications to be taken when the headache is mild in intensity
- Referring appropriate patients to the physician for diagnosis and treatment
- Helping sufferers identify possible triggers.

The nurse can meet headache patients during the course of their regular duties (opportunistically or during health screenings) or by the setting up of a dedicated headache clinic.

7.4   What is the role of the primary care physician?

With the help of these other healthcare professionals, the physician can concentrate at the first visit on:

■ The accurate differential diagnosis of the headache
■ Choosing medications appropriate to the patient's illness severity and lifestyle needs, or
■ Referring patients with sinister symptoms, short, sharp headache, cluster headache, chronic daily headache or some facial pain syndromes to a specialist.

At follow-up visits, the physician can:

■ Review the progress of the patient and modify treatment if indicated
■ Refer to specialists those patients who cannot be dealt with in the primary care setting, e.g. those with migraine resistant to acute and/or prophylactic therapy.

7.5   What is the role of the specialist physician?

Not every headache patient can be dealt with successfully in primary care. Many patients with migraine resistant to treatment, cluster headache, chronic daily headache and suspected sinister headaches need to be referred to a specialist physician. Most commonly, the patient is referred to a neurologist or a headache specialist. It is important that the specialist physician acts as a member of the primary care headache team, informing the primary care physician of the diagnosis and treatment choices, as much of the future management of these patients devolves into primary care.

7.6   What is the role of the community nurse?

Community nurses (e.g. school or college nurses, workplace nurses and district nurses) meet people who are conducting their normal activities at work or elsewhere in the community. In these circumstances, patients may complain about headaches spontaneously or the nurse may be able to deduce that the patient has headache from symptoms present. The nurse can either advise the patient on ways to self-manage their headache if it is mild or to see their primary care physician for treatment if it is more severe in intensity.

7.7   What is the role of the optician?

Opticians see many people with headache, many of whom have eye strain and can be successfully treated by a prescription for spectacles. However, they also see people with migraine and other common headaches. The optician can be a useful medical interface for these sufferers and advise them to see their primary care physician if they suspect that eyestrain is not the cause of the headache.

7.8 What is the role of the dentist?

The dentist sees people with jaw and facial pain, some of whom may have forms of headache. A simple understanding of headache diagnosis would allow them to differentiate the patients with jaw pain that they can treat from those with facial pain and headache who are best referred to a physician.

7.9 What is the role of the alternative practitioner?

An increasing number of headache sufferers now go to alternative practitioners as their primary source of medical advice for migraine and other headaches (e.g. chiropractors, osteopaths, herbalists, acupuncturists and homeopathists). This book has illustrated that some alternative therapies may be of value in helping the patient to manage their headaches (see Q 5.64) but they are unlikely to be effective management strategies on their own. It is therefore important that the alternative practitioner ascertains from their patients which medical therapies they use for headache and advises the patient with severe headaches to also attend their primary care physician for care. Treatment does not have to be mutually exclusive – a few patients will cope on alternative therapies alone but most patients using alternative therapies also require prescribed medications.

7.10 What is the role of the patient?

The patient is perhaps the most important member of the primary care headache team, as all activities are sourced from them. The patient needs to:

- Be able to discuss their headache history
- Understand their diagnosis and management plan and what it is likely to achieve
- Agree to the course of therapy
- Be motivated to continue with and monitor their therapy, and return to the clinic for follow-up.

The patient needs medical help to accomplish all these goals. To achieve this they need education and advice from the professional members of the team.

7.11 How does a primary care headache team work?

Figure 7.1 shows a schematic diagram of how a primary care headache team may work in practice. There is a core medical team of the primary care physician, practice nurse and their assistants. Pharmacists, community

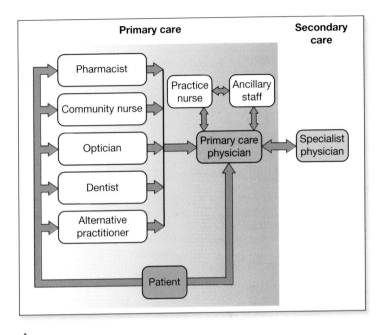

▲

Fig. 7.1 The primary care headache team.

nurses, opticians, dentists and alternative practitioners form associate members of the team.

The patient can access medical care from any member of the team, who will refer them to the primary care physician if necessary. The specialist physician then forms an additional resource for the primary care physician to use where necessary.

Such a team can work without a formal organisation, providing all members are educated about headache and its treatment. In practice, this is often not the case and there is a good argument for a more formal agreement between healthcare professionals on headache care in the community.

For the healthcare professional with an interest in headache, help can be gained from one of the many professional organisations that deal with headache research and treatment (see Appendix 2). Of these, the Migraine Trust, the Migraine in Primary Care Advisors (MIPCA) and the Primary Care Network are perhaps the best source of advice for the primary care headache team internationally, in the UK and in North America, respectively. The International Headache Society, the American Headache

Society and the British Association for the Study of Headache (BASH) are aimed more at the neurologist and headache specialist.

7.12 What are the '10 Commandments' of headache treatment in primary care?

As a memory aid and a stimulus for discussion, I have identified the following '10 Commandments' of headache management. These are not aimed to be comprehensive but, I hope, provide some essential 'dos and don'ts' that will help the healthcare professional to diagnose and manage headache efficiently.

Screening/Diagnosis

1. Almost all headaches are benign and should be managed in general practice.
2. Use questions/a questionnaire assessing impact on daily living for diagnostic screening and to aid management decisions. (Any episodic, high impact headache should be given a default diagnosis of migraine.)

Management

3. Share migraine management between the doctor and patient. (The patient taking control of their management and the doctor providing education and guidance.)
4. Provide individualised care for migraine and encourage patients to treat themselves. (Migraine attacks are highly variable in frequency, duration, symptomatology and impact.)
5. Follow-up patients, preferably with migraine diaries. (Invite the patient to return for further management and apply a proactive policy.)
6. Adapt migraine management to changes that occur in the illness and its presentation over the years. (For example, migraine may change to chronic daily headache over time.)

Treatments

7. Provide acute medication to all migraine patients and recommend it is taken as early as possible in the attack. (Triptans are the most effective acute medications for migraine. Avoid the use of drugs that may cause analgesic-dependent headache, e.g. regular analgesics, codeine and ergotamine.)
8. Prescribe prophylactic medications to patients who have four or more migraine attacks per month or who are resistant to acute medications. (First-line prophylactic medications are beta-blockers, sodium valproate and amitriptyline.)
9. Monitor prophylactic therapy regularly.
10. Ensure that the patient is comfortable with the treatment recommended and that it is practical for their lifestyle and headache presentation.

PATIENT QUESTIONS

7.13 Can a pharmacist treat my migraines?

Pharmacists are key members of the care team for people with migraine. They are knowledgeable about prescription and nonprescription medications and are a good source of information on migraine treatments. Many of them also provide vital links to the doctor. Working with a specific pharmacist who knows the treatments you are taking can prevent many medication problems. They can also provide instructions on the best use of medications, possible side effects and benefits. Pharmacists cannot formally diagnose migraine but have enough general knowledge to provide considerable guidance about migraine care.

7.14 How can the practice nurse help me with my migraine?

The practice nurse is an invaluable source of advice about migraine. She can provide you with lots of information about migraine and you can talk to her about your headache history and symptoms. She can tell you if you should see your doctor about your migraine and can then help you complete any necessary forms, such as headache histories, headache diaries and MIDAS and HIT forms.

You should feel free to talk to the nurse about your migraine either at a special consultation or when you see her at her regular clinics.

7.15 Do I need to see a doctor about migraine?

Some people with mild or infrequent migraine can manage their illness themselves without medical supervision. However, many people who self-manage their migraine are not achieving the best treatment for themselves. Delaying evaluation can lead to considerable lost time and disruption of personal and family life. You should consult your doctor if you have a series of headaches that interfere with your ability to work or enjoy leisure time, despite your best efforts to treat them. Medical consultation should also be considered if you are using any treatment more than three times a month.

Today, more than ever, migraine is a treatable disease. The cornerstone of successful treatment is an accurate diagnosis and a personalised management plan. The use of prescription medications helps most sufferers. Therefore, physicians are key members of the migraine care team.

7.16 Who else can help me with my migraines?

You can receive help for your migraine from many sources. There are several good books written for patients (see references) and many internet sites that also provide valuable information (see Appendix 2).

Other healthcare professionals can also help. Your community nurse, optician, dentist and alternative practitioners can provide advice and sometimes treatment. However, in most cases, they will advise you to consult your doctor for medical care for your migraine.

7.17 How can I help myself to improve my migraines?

The most successful way to control migraines is to establish a two-way relationship between yourself and your doctor. Be willing to assume an active decision-making role, seek out information and try to develop a 'link' with your own nervous system. Investigate the factors that may provoke or prevent your migraine, learn your body's 'early warning system' that communicates when the nervous system is distressed, and treat migraine attacks quickly and effectively with clear goals of success in mind. The best tool to help you accomplish long-term migraine control is a headache calendar/diary that your doctor can provide.

Future developments in migraine management

8

8.1 What are the current hot topics in migraine research?

There are currently several ongoing initiatives to improve migraine diagnosis and management in the clinic, including:

- Evidence-based guidelines for headache management in primary care
- Impact-based recognition of migraine rather than formal diagnostic procedures
- Phase-specific treatment of migraine
- New migraine therapies in development.

These initiatives are in varying stages of development and implementation and should be introduced into specialist and general clinical practice over the next few years.

8.2 What new guidelines for migraine management are desirable?

Primary care is unique among medical specialities and requires its own set of management tools. For example, primary care physicians work under greater demands to evaluate more patients in a shorter time span than do most specialists. In the context of primary care, physicians frequently prioritise many divergent patient complaints and at the same time attempt to integrate preventative and health maintenance efforts. Thus, primary care physicians need guidelines that are time-efficient and directed to appropriate decisions of care.

When patients are referred to a consultant they most often present with specific disease complaints. Most efforts to provide clinical guidelines are created by specialists and are pathology-based with a focus on a specific disease state. In this context, clinical guidelines created by specialists are more appropriate for their own method of practice.

Patients entering the medical system at the primary care level often bring multiple concerns and diverse undifferentiated symptomatology. Physicians are required to manage patients, not just specific disease entities. Consequently, guidelines are needed that focus on patient management and the early evolution of disease conditions. They need to focus on early recognition of diseases for which treatment is available and provide clear outcome expectations for patients. As principles of care, guidelines should be instruments to prioritise patients quickly into appropriate management algorithms.

As we have seen earlier in this book, there are several relatively new sets of headache guidelines available, all based on evidence from randomised clinical trials and other sources (*see Qs 5.11–15*). These will form the basis of revised guidelines for use in primary care. Due to different medical practices and available drugs, new guidelines will need to be tailored to individual countries. However, the basic principles of an accurate diagnosis, assessment of patients' illness severity, impact and needs, and provision of appropriate treatment tailored to each patient can be applied to all. The US Headache Consortium guidelines will no doubt be developed further – and the Migraine in Primary Care Advisors (MIPCA) guidelines have been revised, with new guidelines published in the second half of 2002.

8.3 Is a formal headache diagnosis essential?

Studies showing that high impact, episodic headaches usually indicate migraine have led to debate about whether a formal diagnostic procedure is necessary for migraine. Some physicians have proposed that low-impact headaches should be treated with analgesics and high-impact headaches with migraine-specific medications without further investigation. Diagnosis is reserved for those patients who fail on the initial medications prescribed.

Of course, this procedure flies in the face of normal clinical practice, where diagnosis precedes and drives the treatment given. However, the general principles are sound and have been used to simplify migraine diagnosis in primary care from the unwieldy and relatively complex International Headache Society (IHS) diagnostic criteria. The MIPCA diagnostic scheme uses questions based on headache impact to diagnose migraine from other headache disorders and aims to diagnose all major headaches in four questions, with additional investigations necessary for sinister headaches and short-lasting chronic headaches (*see Q 3.7 and Fig. 3.1*).

The equally daring impact-based recognition of migraine scheme of the US Primary Care Network also incorporates an impact question and aims to diagnose the headache type using only four questions (*see Q 8.4*). Both these schemes are simple to use and very practical for primary care, although they perhaps should be used together with other investigations to confirm the diagnosis. Further research into the MIPCA and Primary Care Network schemes should lead to more accurate but simple diagnostic questionnaires for use in primary care.

8.4 What is impact-based recognition of migraine?

The rationale for an impact-based recognition scheme is that the medical relevance of migraine is largely related to the degree of disruption migraine produces for a given sufferer. This in turn is the major determinant of treatment need. The impact-based recognition scheme of the US Primary Care Network consists of four questions:

1. Do your headaches interfere with your ability to work or engage in family and social functions?
2. Has the pattern of your headache changed over the last 6 months?

3. How frequently do you have any kind of headaches?
4. What are you doing to treat your headaches?

The first question quickly separates medically relevant headaches from those more trivial in nature. Migraine should be considered the default diagnosis for headache that significantly interferes with a person's ability to function. Examining how function is disrupted allows the physician to assess treatment needs and creates rapport with the patient. A positive response necessitates questions on migraine-specific associations, such as the presence of nausea, sensory sensitivity, positive family history, and in women, menstrual association.

The second question is designed to alert the physician to sinister headache conditions. A new or different headache mandates a thorough diagnostic approach, while a stable headache pattern provides reassurance to the physician and patient.

The third question alerts the physician to chronic headache patterns. In turn, this relates to consideration of prophylactic medications and tempers the use of acute treatment medications.

The fourth question screens for medication overuse and the effectiveness of self-treatment efforts.

Impact-based recognition is a time-efficient screening method that allows providers to quickly screen patients for headache in the outpatient setting, even when they are being evaluated for other complaints.

8.5 What is phase-specific treatment for migraine?

Targeting specific migraine treatment to the phase of the illness is another relatively new concept from the US Primary Care Network. We have reviewed this strategy briefly earlier in the book (*see* Q 5.55). Therapy can be targeted at the prodrome, aura, headache and postheadache phases (*Fig. 8.1*).

TREATMENT DURING THE PRODROME

During the premonitory period, simply removing oneself from stressful environments or engaging in relaxation or biofeedback can often abort the impending migraine. Some preliminary studies indicate that acute treatments such as naratriptan, DHE and NSAIDs may be effective when taken during the prodrome.

TREATMENT DURING THE MIGRAINE AURA

Many therapies have been suggested to treat aura but none has clear evidence of efficacy. For example, there is little evidence for the efficacy of triptans when taken during the aura period. However, if simple auras are consistently followed by headache, treatment with oral drugs can be initiated to prevent the unnecessary delay of waiting for the headache.

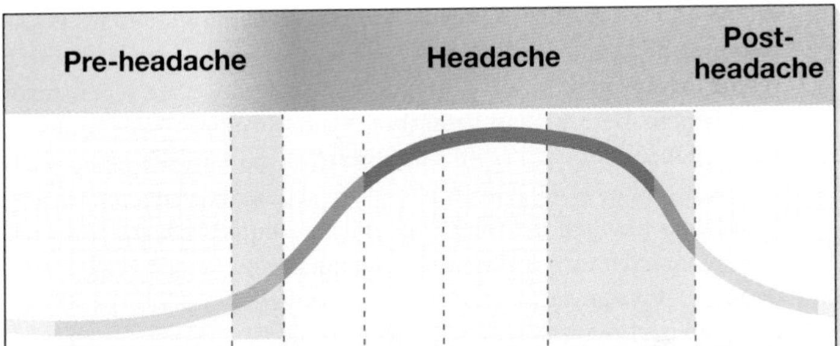

	Pre-headache		Headache			Post-headache
	Prodrome	Aura	Mild	Moderate	Severe	Rescue	Postdrome
Triptans (oral, nasal)	+/++		++++	+++	++		
Subcut. triptan					++++		
OTCs ASA + paracetamol + caffeine			++		+	++/+++	++
NSAIDs	+		++				++
Isometheptene			++				
Narcotics Phenothiazines						++	
Biofeedback Thermal + relaxation training	+++						

Fig. 8.1 Phase-specific acute therapy for migraine, according to the US Primary Care Network.

TREATMENT DURING THE MILD HEADACHE PHASE

Many headache specialists have encouraged treating headache early. Simple and combination analgesics can be taken before the headache appears if the patient has clear signs of an impending headache. Triptans are now recommended to be taken when the headache is established but mild in intensity. However, this is not a recommended strategy for patients with very frequent headache attacks since it could lead to analgesic overuse.

TREATMENT DURING MODERATE TO SEVERE HEADACHE

Most of the evidence from clinical trials is derived from interventions during the moderate to severe headache phase of migraine. A wide range of drugs have reported efficacy for relieving pain and associated migraine symptoms. The most effective are the triptans but analgesics and antiemetics also have some utility.

TREATMENT USING RESCUE MEDICATION

Occasionally an attack of migraine may not respond to initial therapeutic interventions. In order to prevent unnecessary utilisation of healthcare resources and provide relief, it is often wise to provide patients with a rescue therapy in advance. Commonly used products are subcutaneous sumatriptan, butorphanol nasal spray *(not available in Europe)* and parenteral phenothiazines. It is important to monitor the frequency of use of rescue therapies. In general, if patients require rescue more than once or twice a month, then first-line acute therapy should be adjusted, efforts to initiate interventions earlier in the migraine process encouraged, and/or the addition of prophylactic medications instituted. In addition, coping strategies and resources of the patient should be assessed.

TREATMENT DURING THE POSTHEADACHE PHASE

Many patients report that they experience significant impact from migraine in the postheadache period. Little formal study has been given to this phase of migraine but, in general, simple analgesics and NSAIDs improve symptoms. Re-hydration is also recommended.

Phase-specific treatment can be an effective strategy for many patients with migraine. It encourages their vigilance and participation in treatment. It also affords the opportunity to intervene early and with specific efforts. This, in many patients, limits the impact of migraine and reduces treatment failures.

8.6 What new headache treatments are in development?

Several new medications for migraine and other headaches are in development and at least some will be introduced into clinical practice over the next few years. Treatment modalities under investigation include:

- New triptans, some with novel mechanisms of action
- The combination of a triptan with an analgesic (e.g. an NSAID) or an antiemetic to improve gastric motility has the potential to provide synergistic effects on migraine pain and associated symptoms over and above that provided by the triptan alone
- The co-administration of a long half-life triptan (e.g. naratriptan) together with a faster-acting triptan (e.g. sumatriptan) has potential for the treatment of patients who frequently report headache recurrence following triptan therapy
- Medications designed to inhibit the sterile neurogenic inflammation associated with migraine pathogenesis but which do not have significant vasoconstrictor effects. These drugs are hypothesised to be safer than the triptans, as they will have no significant cardiovascular effects
- Drugs that inhibit the nitric oxide synthase enzyme reduce the level of nitric oxide and so inhibit the development of migraine attacks triggered by this compound

■ Glutamate receptor antagonists show great potential as new acute treatments for migraine
■ New prophylactic medications are also being developed, including botulinum toxin type A (Botox), tizanidine, montelukast and rofecoxib.

8.7 What new triptans are in development?

Despite the huge success of the triptans as acute treatments for migraine, several drugs in this class have failed to make it to market, either due to lack of efficacy or safety concerns:

■ Avitriptan and BMS-181885 – Avitriptan is selective for 5-HT 1B and 1D receptors while BMS-181885 is more potent at the 5-HT 1B receptor. Avitriptan was shown to be an effective acute treatment for migraine but development of both drugs was halted due to concerns over liver toxicity.
■ Alniditan is a potent 5-HT$_{1B/1D}$ agonist that was shown to be an effective and well tolerated acute treatment for migraine but was discontinued when it showed no benefit over sumatriptan.

Several new third-generation triptans are currently in clinical development:

■ IS-159 is a selective and potent 5-HT$_{1B/1D}$ agonist that is being developed in a nasal spray formulation. Phase 2 clinical data showed it was significantly more effective than placebo as an acute treatment for migraine with a 2-hour response rate similar to those reported for nasal spray sumatriptan and zolmitriptan (*see Qs 4.37 and 4.51*). A total of 71% of patients receiving IS-159 reported headache relief at 2 hours compared to 35% receiving placebo.
■ F-11356 is perhaps the most potent of the 5-HT$_{1B/1D}$ agonists in vitro but to date no clinical data have been reported for this product.

8.8 What data are available on combination medications using triptans?

Some preliminary studies have compared the efficacy of triptans given alone or in concert with the antiemetic metoclopramide, NSAIDs or COX-2 inhibitors. The latter two drugs have longer half-lives than the triptans and were hypothesised to reduce the rate of headache recurrence reported with triptans alone:

■ In migraine patients who were nonresponsive to triptans, the combination of sumatriptan 50 mg and metoclopramide 10 mg was more effective than sumatriptan 50 mg alone. Headache relief after

2 hours was reported by 19% of patients in the combination group compared to 3% in the sumatriptan only group.

■ The combination of naratriptan 2.5 mg and the NSAID naproxen 500 mg was shown to be more effective than naratriptan 2.5 mg alone in terms of higher headache relief rates after 2 hours (54% vs 40%) and 4 hours (70% vs 58%) and lower headache recurrence (11% vs 31%).

■ The combination of sumatriptan 100 mg and the COX-2 inhibitor rofecoxib 25 mg was not more effective than sumatriptan 100 mg alone in terms of headache relief, but the rate of recurrence was lower (26% vs 44%) and the time to recurrence longer (14 h vs 10 h) in the combination group.

■ The combination of rizatriptan 10 mg and the COX-2 inhibitor rofecoxib 25 mg was numerically, but not significantly, more effective than rizatriptan 10 mg alone in terms of complete headache relief – but the rate of recurrence was significantly lower (20% vs 53%) in the combination group.

These results indicate that the addition of an antiemetic, an NSAID or a COX-2 inhibitor to a triptan may all be superior to the triptan alone, particularly for groups of patients who respond suboptimally to the triptans. However, these results must be confirmed in large controlled clinical studies before this strategy can be recommended in clinical practice.

8.9 What data are available on medications designed to inhibit sterile neurogenic inflammation?

In the search for new acute medications for migraine, the holy grail is a drug that is as effective as the triptans, but has no vasoconstrictor activity, and so is not associated with the risk of cardiovascular side effects. The idea is to inhibit the sterile neurogenic inflammation, but not the vasodilatation, that is involved with migraine pathogenesis (*see Q 2.41*). Substance P antagonists, endothelin antagonists, nonvasoconstricting 5-HT 1D agonists and conformationally-restricted analogues of sumatriptan and zolmitriptan have all been tried but found ineffective.

At face value, these results would indicate that the inhibition of neurogenic inflammation is not effective on its own to abort migraine and that vasoconstriction is also necessary. However, data on the selective 5-HT_{1F} agonist LY334370 and a new CGRP antagonist gave promising results, suggesting that the original hypothesis may still be valid. The end result of all this research is that the concept of neural inflammation as a sole target for migraine therapy is not proven. New therapies targeting this mechanism will not be available for the foreseeable future and remain for the present in the research domain only.

8.10   What nitric oxide synthase inhibitors are in development?

Nitric oxide is a small, membrane-permeable, lipophilic gas that can act as a neuronal messenger. Several pieces of evidence implicate it as a key trigger of migraine attacks (*see Q 2.44*). Nitric oxide is synthesised by the nitric oxide synthase enzyme, which is now a target for acute treatments. A nitric oxide synthase inhibitor has been produced (546C88) and a preliminary study conducted with it. 546C88 was shown to be significantly more effective than placebo as an acute treatment for migraine. Of 15 patients studied, 67% reported headache relief after 2 hours with 546C88, compared to 14% receiving placebo ($P < 0.05$). However, the response to 546C88 was not sustained much beyond the 2-hour endpoint.

Although promising, these data are very preliminary. Much more work needs to be done before even the principle of this approach for migraine treatment can be established. Therapies for use in the clinic are a long way off.

8.11   What glutamate receptor antagonists are in development?

Glutamate may be involved in migraine pathogenesis. Glutamic acid, glutamine, glycine, cysteic acid and homocysteic acids are all elevated above normal levels in migraine sufferers, and even more so during an attack. Glutamate receptors are located in the trigeminal ganglion, localised on the same neurons as 5-HT 1B, 1D and 1F receptors. Antagonists of glutamate receptors are therefore potential acute treatments for migraine. One such compound (LY293558) has been synthesised and is an antagonist at the AMPA and KA glutamate receptor subtypes.

A small placebo-controlled study has compared the response to intravenous LY293558 with that to subcutaneous sumatriptan 6 mg for the acute treatment of migraine. At 2 hours after treatment, 87% of patients receiving sumatriptan, 69% receiving LY293558 and 25% receiving placebo reported headache relief. Both active treatments were significantly superior to placebo ($P < 0.01$). This treatment strategy is therefore extremely promising and the results from further clinical trials of glutamate antagonists are eagerly anticipated. However, therapies for clinical use are several years away.

8.12   What new prophylactic medications are in development?

Improvements over the past decade in acute therapies for migraine have not been matched by the development of new prophylactic medications. These are urgently needed, as existing therapies exhibit suboptimal efficacy and are associated with many side effects. Much of the present research in this field involves new-generation anticonvulsants such as topiramate, levetiracetam and lamotrigine. There is also a new calcium channel antagonist, an angiotensin converting enzyme inhibitor and an inhibitor of cortical spreading depression in development. Perhaps the most promising new therapies are:

- Botulinum toxin type A (Botox)
- The alpha-2-adrenergic agonist tizanidine
- The leukotriene receptor antagonist montelukast (used as adjunctive therapy in the treatment of asthma)
- The COX-2 inhibitor rofecoxib (used for arthritis).

These four compounds have all shown positive results in initial studies conducted for migraine prophylaxis. These results indicate that, finally, there may be some new and more effective prophylactic agents for migraine on the horizon, although they all require further studies to confirm their clinical profiles.

8.13 What is the future of migraine care?

In many ways the 1990s were the golden age for migraine, with new understanding of its aetiology and pathogenesis and the development of the triptans, which have revolutionised acute treatment. The end result is that, today, migraine is probably the most successfully managed neurological disease. Triptans are likely to remain the gold standard for migraine treatment for several years to come, as new acute and prophylactic treatments are unlikely to become available in the near future. The challenge for today is to transfer the recent very real treatment advances for migraine into the primary care setting, where patients are still managed suboptimally.

Primary care provides the foundation and platform from which headache care will advance clinically. Primary care has much to offer today for those patients suffering from migraine. I hope that this book provides the information and strategies that will help the primary care physician to manage migraine and other headaches more efficiently in their practice.

APPENDIX 1
Antimigraine drugs

ACUTE TREATMENTS: *Analgesics*

Drug (generic name)	Route of administration	Trade name	Formulation	Dose(s)	Side effects	Comments
Tolfenamic acid	Oral	Clotam Rapid (UK)	Tablet 200 mg	1–2 times per attack	GI upset Skin reactions Dysuria	NSAID Rarely causes reversible liver function changes Licensed in UK for migraine
Ibuprofen	Oral		Tablet 200, 400, 600, 800 mg	800 mg then q 8 hours PRN	GI upset/ haemorrhage Rash Thrombo-cytopenia	NSAID Approved in USA for OTC use
Naproxen	Oral	Naprosyn (UK, USA)	Tablet 250, 375, 500 mg	250–500 mg then q 8 hours PRN	Rash GI intolerance Headache, tinnitus, vertigo Blood, renal, hepatic disorders	NSAID
Ketoprofen	Oral	Ketocid (UK)	Tablet 25, 50, 75 mg	75–100 mg then q 6–8 hours PRN	GI intolerance CNS effects	NSAID
Meclofenamate	Oral		Tablet 100 mg	100 mg then q 8 hours PRN	GI intolerance	NSAID

ACUTE TREATMENTS: *Combination analgesics*

Drug (generic name)	Route of administration	Trade name	Formulation	Dose(s)	Side effects	Comments
Paracetamol*/ Domperidone	Oral	Domperamol (UK)	Tablet 500 mg/ 10 mg	2–8 tablets per attack	Raised serum prolactin Galactorrhoea Gynaecomastia Reduced libido Rash Allergic reactions	Analgesic/ Antidopaninergic Rarely causes extrapyramidal symptoms Not available in USA
Isometheptene/ Paracetamol*	Oral	Midrid (UK/USA)	Capsule 65 mg/325 mg	2–5 capsules per attack	Dizziness	Sympathomimetic/ Analgesic
Isometheptene/ Dichloralphenazone/ Paracetamol*	Oral	Midrin (USA)	Capsule 65 mg/ 100 mg/ 325 mg	2–5 capsules per attack	Dizziness Skin rash	Sympathomimetic/ Analgesic Not available in UK
Aspirin/ Metoclopramide	Oral	Migramax (UK)	Powder in sachets 900 mg/10 mg	1–3 sachets per attack	GI upset and haemorrhage Drowsiness Endocrine disorders Extrapyramidal symptoms	Analgesic/Antiemetic
Paracetamol*/ Metoclopramide	Oral	Paramax (UK)	Tablets 500 mg/5 mg	2–6 tablets per attack	Extrapyramidal symptoms Raised serum prolactin Drowsiness Diarrhoea	Analgesic/Antiemetic
Paracetamol*/ Aspirin/caffeine	Oral	Excedrin (USA)	Tablets 325 mg/326 mg/65 mg	2–8 tablets per attack		OTC analgesic combination Licensed for mild to moderate migraine in the USA Not available in UK

*Paracetamol is known as acetaminophen in the USA

ACUTE TREATMENTS: *Monotherapy and combinations including opiate analgesics*

Drug (generic name)	Route of administration	Trade name	Formulation	Dose(s)	Side effects	Comments
Buclizine/ Paracetamol*/ Codeine	Oral	Migraleve (UK)	Pink tablets: 6.25 mg/ 500 mg/8 mg Yellow tablets: 0 mg/500 mg/ 8 mg	Two pink tablets at onset plus up to six yellow tablets per attack	Drowsiness	Simple and opiate analgesic/ Antiemetic No available in USA
Butalbital/Aspirin/ Caffeine/Codeine	Oral	Fiorinol (USA)	50 mg/ 325 mg/ 40 mg/30mg		Sedation Risk of rebound and medication overuse	Barbiturate/Simple and opiate analgesic Not available in UK
Butorphanol	Nasal spray	Stadol (USA)	Nasal spray 1 mg	1 spray, may be repeated after 1 hour: sequence may be repeated 4 hours after last dose	Dizziness Drowsiness Nausea/vomiting Vertigo Blurred vision Nervousness Taste perversion	Opiate analgesic Primary role in rescue Not available in UK
Hydromorphone	Suppository		Suppository 3 mg	1–2 suppositories per attack	Constipation Nausea/vomiting Drowsiness Dependence Overuse Impairment of function	Opiate analgesic Primary role in rescue Not licensed for migraine in UK

*Paracetamol is known as acetaminophen in the USA

ACUTE TREATMENTS: *Triptans*

Drug (generic name)	Route of administration	Trade name	Formulation	Dose(s)	Side effects	Comments
Almotriptan	Oral	Almogran (UK) Axert (USA)	Tablet 6.25 mg, 12.5 mg	1–2 12.5 mg tablets per attack	Dizziness Somnolence GI upset Fatigue	
Sumatriptan	Oral	Imigran (UK) Imitrex (USA)	Tablet 25 mg, 50 mg, 100 mg	50 mg or 100 mg (1–3 doses per attack) Maximum 300 mg per attack in UK and 200 mg in USA	Pain Heaviness/pressure Fatigue Dizziness Drowsiness Weakness Increases in BP	
Sumatriptan	Nasal spray	Imigran (UK) Imitrex (USA)	Nasal spray 5 mg, 20 mg	1–2 20 mg doses per attack	Bitter taste Pain Heaviness/pressure Fatigue Dizziness Drowsiness Weakness Increases in BP	
Sumatriptan	Subcutaneous injection	Imigran (UK) Imitrex (USA)	Subcutaneous injection 6 mg	1–2 6 mg doses per attack, separated by at least 1 hour	Pain at injection site Pain Heaviness/pressure Fatigue Dizziness Drowsiness Weakness Increases in BP	

ACUTE TREATMENTS: *Triptans (cont'd)*

Drug (generic name)	Route of administration	Trade name	Formulation	Dose(s)	Side effects	Comments
Rizatriptan	Oral	Maxalt (UK, USA)	Tablet 5 mg, 10 mg	1–2 10 mg doses per attack in the UK 1–3 doses per 24 hours separated by at least 2 hours in the USA	Dizziness Somnolence Asthenia Abdominal/Chest pain Palpitations Tachycardia GI upset Musculoskeletal symptoms CNS disturbances Pharyngeal discomfort Dyspnoea Pruritus Sweating Urticaria Blurred vision Hot flushes Tongue swelling Rash Toxic epidermal necrolysis Bad taste	
Rizatriptan	Oral	Maxalt Melt	Orally disintegrating tablet 10 mg	1–2 10 mg doses per attack in the UK 1–3 doses per 24 hours separated by at least 2 hours in the USA	See above for Maxalt	

ACUTE TREATMENTS: *Triptans (cont'd)*

Drug (generic name)	Route of administration	Trade name	Formulation	Dose(s)	Side effects	Comments
Naratriptan	Oral	Naramig (UK) Amerge (USA)	Tablet 1.0 mg, 2.5 mg	1–2 2.5 mg doses per attack in the UK 1.0–2.5 mg: may be repeated after 4 hours up to 5 mg per 24 hours in the USA	Malaise Fatigue Dizziness Nausea Pain, warmth, heaviness or pressure in any part of the body (including the throat and chest) Bradycardia Tachycardia Visual disturbance	
Eletriptan	Oral	Relpax (UK, USA)	Tablet 20, 40 80 mg	Unknown at present		Not available yet in UK and USA
Zolmitriptan	Oral	Zomig (UK, USA)	Tablet 2.5 mg	1–3 2.5 mg doses per attack (can increase dose to 5 mg if 2.5 mg inadequate (maximum 15 mg per attack in the UK Doses separated by at least 2 hours and maximum 24-hour dose is 10 mg in the USA	Nausea Dizziness Warm sensation Asthenia Dry mouth Somnolence Heaviness or pressure in throat, neck, limbs or chest Myalgia Muscle weakness Paraesthesia	

ACUTE TREATMENTS: *Triptans (cont'd)*

Drug (generic name)	Route of administration	Trade name	Formulation	Dose(s)	Side effects	Comments
Zolmitriptan	Oral	Zomig Melt	Orally disintegrating tablet 2.5 mg	1–3 2.5 mg doses per attack (can increase dose to 5 mg if 2.5 mg inadequate (maximum 15 mg per attack) in the UK Doses separated by at least 2 hours and maximum 24-hour dose is 10 mg in the USA	See above for Zomig	

ACUTE TREATMENTS: *Ergots*

Drug (generic name)	Route of administration	Trade name	Formulation	Dose(s)	Side effects	Comments
Ergotamine/ Caffeine	Oral	Cafergot	Tablet 1 mg/100 mg	1–4 tablets per attack (maximum 8 tablets per week)	Nausea Vomiting Abdominal pain Circulatory impairment Precordial pain Myocardial ischaemia and infarction Paraesthesia Pleural or retroperitoneal fibrosis	Not available in UK
Ergotamine/ Caffeine	Rectal	Cafergot	Suppository 2 mg/100 mg	1–2 tablets per attack (maximum 4 tablets per week)	See above for oral Cafergot	Not available in UK
Ergotamine/ Cyclizine/Caffeine	Oral	Migril (UK)	Tablets 2 mg/50 mg/ 100 mg	1–4 tablets per attack (maximum 6 tablets per week)	See above for oral Cafergot	Available in UK
Ergotamine	Oral			2 mg	See above for oral Cafergot	Not available in UK
Ergostine/Caffeine		Ergostat (USA)			See above for oral Cafergot	Not available in UK

ACUTE TREATMENTS: *Ergots (cont'd)*

Drug (generic name)	Route of administration	Trade name	Formulation	Dose(s)	Side effects	Comments
Dihydroergotamine	Subcutaneous injection		Subcutaneous injection 1 mg		Nausea/vomiting Dysphoria Flushing Restlessness Anxiety	Not available in UK
Dihydroergotamine	Intramuscular injection	DHE 45 Injection	Intramuscular injection		See above for sc injection	Not available in UK
Dihydroergotamine	Nasal spray	Migranal (USA)	Nasal spray 0.5 mg	4 sprays per attack (2 mg). Maximum 8 sprays per week (4 mg)	Taste alteration Dizziness Drowsiness Nasal inflammation Nausea Sore throat Vomiting Diarrhoea Dry mouth Fatigue Hot flushes Loss of strength Sinus inflammation Stiffness Tingling	Not available in UK

ACUTE TREATMENTS: *Anti-emetics*

Drug (generic name)	Route of administration	Trade name	Formulation	Dose(s)	Side effects	Comments
Prochlorperazine	IM, IV injections Suppository			IM/IV 10 mg Suppository 25 mg	CNS disturbances Anticholinergic effects Akathesia ECG and endocrine changes	Phenothiazine Licensed for nausea and vomiting, but used in migraine adjunctively or as a single agent Often used for rescue
Chlorpromazine	IV injection			IV 12.5 mg	CNS disturbances Sedation Akathesia	Phenothiazine Licensed for nausea and vomiting, but used in migraine adjunctively or as a single agent Often used for rescue

PROPHYLACTIC TREATMENTS: *Beta-blockers*

Drug (generic name)	Route of administration	Trade name	Formulation	Dose(s)	Side effects	Comments
Propranolol	Oral	Beta-Prograne (UK)	Sustained release capsule 160 mg	20–160 mg daily	Cold extremities CNS and sleep disturbances Bradycardia Exertional tiredness Bronchospasm Heart failure Hypotension GI upset Alopecia Thrombocytopenia Dry eyes/skin rash	Noncardioselective beta-blocker
		Inderal LA (UK)	Sustained release capsule 160 mg			
		Syprol (UK)	Oral solution 40 mg			
Metoprolol	Oral	Betaloc (UK) Lopresor (UK)	Tablets 50 mg/100 mg Tablets 50 mg/100 mg	50–200 mg daily	See propranolol above	Cardioselective beta-blocker
Timolol	Oral	Betim (UK)	Tablets 10 mg	10–20 mg daily	See propranolol above	Noncardioselective beta-blocker
Nadolol	Oral	Corgard (UK)	Tablets 40 mg/80 mg	80–160 mg daily	See propranolol above	Noncardioselective beta-blocker
Atenolol	Oral		Tablets	25–100 mg daily	See propranolol above	Available in USA, but not in UK

PROPHYLACTIC TREATMENTS: *5-HT$_2$ antagonists*

Drug (generic name)	Route of administration	Trade name	Formulation	Dose(s)	Side effects	Comments
Methysergide	Oral	Deseril (UK) Sansert (USA)	Tablets 1 mg, 2 mg	1–3 times daily (UK) 2–8 mg daily (USA)	Inflammatory fibrosis Arterial spasm Nausea Vomiting Heartburn Abdominal discomfort Lassitude Oedema Leg cramps Dizziness Drowsiness Weight gain Skin eruptions Hair loss CNS disturbances	Serotonin antagonist
Cyproheptadine	Oral	Periactin (UK)	Tablets 4 mg	1 every 4–6 hours	Drowsiness Impaired reactions Anticholinergic effects Weight gain	Antihistamine/ Serotonin antagonist Not recommended
Pizotifen	Oral	Sanomigran (UK)	Tablets 0.5 mg/1.5 mg Elixir 0.25 mg/5 mL	Normally 1.5 mg daily (maximum 4.5 mg daily)	Drowsiness Increased appetite Weight gain	Serotonin antagonist Not available in USA
Lisuride	Oral			0.075 mg to 0.15 mg per day	Sedation Nausea Dizziness	Not available in UK and USA

PROPHYLACTIC TREATMENTS: *Other prophylactic drugs*

Drug (generic name)	Route of administration	Trade name	Formulation	Dose(s)	Side effects	Comments
Clonidine	Oral and transcutaneous patch (USA only)	Dixarit (UK) Clonadine (USA) Catapres patch (USA)	Tablets 25 micrograms (UK) Tablets/patch 0.1, 0.2, 0.3 mg (USA)	2–3 tablets morning and evening (UK) 1 tablet morning and evening or 1 patch weekly (USA)	Sedation Dry mouth Dizziness Sleeplessness	Central alpha-agonist Not recommended
Divalproex sodium	Oral	Depakote (USA)	Tablets 125 mg/ 250 mg/ 500 mg	125–1,000 mg daily	Liver damage Abdominal pain Abnormal thinking Breathing difficulty Bronchitis, Bruising Constipation Diarrhoea, Dizziness Emotional changes Fever/flu symptoms Hair loss, Headache Indigestion, Infection Insomnia Appetite loss Memory loss Nasal inflammation Nausea/vomiting Ringing in the ears Sleepiness Sore throat, Tremor Vision problems Weakness Weight gain	Anticonvulsant Licensed for migraine in the USA, but not UK Teratogenic

PROPHYLACTIC TREATMENTS: *Other prophylactic drugs (cont'd)*

Drug (generic name)	Route of administration	Trade name	Formulation	Dose(s)	Side effects	Comments
Amitriptyline	Oral	Elavil (USA) Lentizol/ Triptafen (UK)	Tablets 10, 25, 50, 75, 100, 150 mg	10–100 mg per day (maximum 200 mg per day)	Anticholinergic effects (e.g. dry mouth) Constipation Urinary retention Vision changes Palpitations and tachycardia Tinnitus Orthostatic hypotension CNS and neuromuscular effects Gastric irritation Weight changes Allergic skin reactions Jaundice and blood disorders Conduction defects and cardiac arrhythmias Endocrine effects (e.g. changes in libido) Impotence Gynaecomastia and galactorrhoea Changes in blood sugar concentration Mania or schizophrenic symptoms Withdrawal symptoms	Tricyclic antidepressant Licensed for depression, but not migraine, in the UK Other tricyclic antidepressants used in the USA include: Nortriptyline (10–150 mg/day) Protriptyline (5–30 mg/day)

PROPHYLACTIC TREATMENTS: *Other prophylactic drugs (cont'd)*

Drug (generic name)	Route of administration	Trade name	Formulation	Dose(s)	Side effects	Comments
Fluoxetine	Oral	Prozac (UK/USA)	Capsule	20 mg every other day to 40 mg daily	Insomnia Fatigue Tremor Stomach pain	SSRI Licensed for depression, but not migraine, in the UK
Flunarizine	Oral			5–10 mg per day	Sedation Weight gain Depression Tremor Parkinsonism	Calcium channel blocker Not licensed for migraine prevention in UK and USA
Nimodipine	Oral			120 mg per day	Abdominal discomfort	Calcium channel blocker Not licensed for migraine prevention in the UK
Verapamil	Oral			80–360 mg per day	Constipation	Calcium channel blocker Not licensed for migraine prevention in the UK
Dihydroergotamine				2–3 mg per day	Nausea Headache Dizziness Development of CDH	Ergot alkaloid Not licensed for migraine prevention in UK and USA
Naproxen	Oral	Naprosyn (UK, USA)		500 mg per day	Dyspepsia GI bleeding Constipation Tinnitus Bronchospasm	NSAID Not licensed for migraine prevention in the UK

PROPHYLACTIC TREATMENTS: *Other prophylactic drugs (cont'd)*

Drug (generic name)	Route of administration	Trade name	Formulation	Dose(s)	Side effects	Comments
Aspirin	Oral			250 mg per day	See naproxen above	Not licensed for migraine prevention in the UK
Oestradiol	Percutaneous gel		Percutaneous gel	15 mg per day for 7 days during menstruation		Short-term prevention of migraine associated with menses

APPENDIX 2
Useful addresses and websites for the GP and the patient

FOR THE PRIMARY CARE PHYSICIAN

Societies, journals and congresses

International Headache Society (IHS)

www.i-h-s.org

Journal: *Cephalalgia*
Congress: International Headache Congress (biannual)

American Headache Society (AHS)

19 Mantua Road
Mt. Royal
NJ 08061
USA
Tel.: (+1) 856 423 0043
Fax: (+1) 856 423 0082
E-mail: ahshq@talley.com
www.ahsnet.org

Journal: *Headache*
Congress: American Headache Society Meeting (annual)

Migraine in Primary Care Advisors (MIPCA)

Maggie Adams (Secretary)
Woodstock
Tilford Road
Hindhead
Surrey
GU26 6SF
UK
Tel.: (+44) (0)1428 607 837
www.mipca.org.uk

Primary Care Network

1230 E. Kingsley Street – Suite G
Springfield
MO 65804
USA
Tel.: (+1) 417 886 2026
Fax: (+1) 417 883 7476
www.primarycarenet.org

British Association for the Study of Headache (BASH)
Carol Taylor (secretariat)
Wood Dene
Stanton Lees, nr. Matlock
Derbyshire
DE4 2LQ
UK
Tel.: +44 (0) 1629 733 406
E-mail: carol@caroltaylor.co.uk
www.bash.org.uk

The Migraine Trust
45 Great Ormond Street
London
WC1N 3HZ
UK
Tel.: +44 (0) 207 831 4818
Fax: +44 (0) 207 831 5174
E-mail: via the website
www.migrainetrust.org
Congress: Migraine Trust International Symposium (biannual)

Websites other than the above containing useful information

Medscape
www.neurology.medscape.com

Doctor's Guide Migraine Site
www.pslgroup.com/migraine.htm

MIDAS website
www.migraine-disability.net

HIT websites
www.amIhealthy.com
www.headachetest.com

FOR THE PATIENT

Societies

World Headache Alliance (WHA)

3288 Old Coach Road
Burlington
Ontario
Canada
L7N 3P7
E-mail: info@w-h-a.org
www.w-h-a.org

Migraine Trust

(see above)

National Headache Foundation (NHF)

428 W. St. James Place
2nd Floor
Chicago
IL 60614-2750
USA
Tel.: (+1) 888 643 5552
E-mail: info@headaches.org
www.headaches.org

American Council for Headache Education (ACHE)

19 Mantua Road
Mount Royal
NJ 08061
USA
Tel.: (+1) 856 423 0258
E-mail: acheq@talley.com
www.achenet.org

Migraine Action Association (UK)

Unit 6
Oakley Hay Lodge Business Park
Great Folds Road
Great Oakley
Northants
NN18 9AS
UK
Tel.: +44 (0) 1536 461 333

Fax: +44 (0) 1536 461 444
E-mail: info@migraine.org.uk
www.migraine.org.uk

Websites other than the above containing useful information

Health Destinations – Headache Site
www.connect2health.com

Primary Care Network – Headache Site
www.headachecare.com

Ronda's Migraine Page Site
www.migrainepage.com

MIDAS website
www.migraine-disability.net

HIT websites
www.amIhealthy.com
www.headachetest.com

REFERENCES

The following references have proved invaluable sources of information for this book. The 'specialist sources' section provides in depth information on general and specific topics. The 'material for the primary care physician' section provides more general information aimed at the primary care physician. The 'material for the patient' provides easy to read material for the patient.

SPECIALIST SOURCES

Breslau N, Rasmussen BK. The impact of migraine: Epidemiology, risk factors, and co-morbidities. *Neurology* 2001; **56** (Suppl 1): 4–12.

Campbell JK, Penzien DB, Wall EM. Evidenced-based guidelines for migraine headache: behavioural and physical treatments. *Neurology* 2000; **54** www.aan.com/public/practiceguidelines/04.pdf

Diener HC, Limmroth V. The management of migraine. *Rev Contemp Pharmacother* 1994; **5**: 271–84.

Dowson AJ. Assessing the impact of migraine. *Curr Med Res Opin* 2001; **17**: 298–309.

Edmeads J, Láinez JM, Brandes JL et al. Potential of the Migraine Disability Assessment (MIDAS) Questionnaire as a public health initiative and in clinical practice. *Neurology* 2001; **56** (Suppl 1):S29–34.

Ferrari MD. The economic burden of migraine to society. *Pharmacoeconomics* 1998; **13**: 667–76.

Ferrari MD, Roon KI, Lipton RB et al. Oral triptans (serotonin 5-HT$_{1B/1D}$ agonists) in acute migraine treatment: a meta-analysis of 53 trials. *Lancet* 2001; **358**: 1668–75.

Fox AW. Comparative tolerability of oral 5-HT$_{1B/1D}$ agonists. *Headache* 2000; **40**: 521–7.

Headache Classification Committee of the International Headache Society. Classification and diagnostic criteria for headache disorders, cranial neuralgias and facial pain. *Cephalalgia* 1988; **8** (Suppl 7): 19–28.

Lipton RB, Silberstein SD. The role of headache-related disability in migraine management. *Neurology* 2001; **56** (Suppl 1): S35–42.

Matchar DB, Young WB, Rosenberg JH et al. Multispecialty consensus on diagnosis and treatment of headache: pharmacological management of acute attacks. *Neurology* 2000; **54** www.aan.com/public/practiceguidelines/03.pdf

Matharu M, Goadsby PJ. Cluster headache: update on a common neurological problem. *Pract Neurol* 2001; **1**: 42–9.

Mathew NT. Pathophysiology, epidemiology, and impact of migraine. *Clin Cornerstone* 2001; **4**: 1–17.

Olesen J, Tfelt-Hansen P, Welch KMA, eds. *The headaches*, 2nd Edition. New York: Lippincott Williams & Wilkins; 2000.

Peatfield RC, Goadsby PJ, Silberstein SD eds. Drug therapy for migraine. *Curr Med Res Opin* 2001; **17**: Supplement 1.

Ramadan NM, Silberstein SD, Freitag FG et al. Multispecialty consensus on diagnosis and treatment of headache: pharmacological management for prevention of migraine. *Neurology* 2000; **54** www.aan.com/public/practiceguidelines/05.pdf

Sheftell FD, Fox AW. Acute migraine treatment outcome measures: a clinician's view. *Cephalalgia* 2000; **20** (Suppl 2): 14–24.

Silberstein SD, Lipton RB. Chronic daily headache. *Curr Opin Neurol* 2000; **13:** 277–83.

Stewart WF, Lipton RB, Celentano DD et al. Prevalence of migraine headache in the United States. Relation to age, income, race and other sociodemographic factors. *JAMA* 1992; **267:** 64–9.

Stewart WF, Shechter A, Lipton RB. Migraine heterogeneity. Disability, pain intensity, and attack frequency and duration. *Neurology* 1994; **44** (Suppl 4): 24–39.

Tfelt-Hansen P, De Vries P, Saxena PR. Triptans in migraine: a comparative review of pharmacology, pharmacokinetics and efficacy. *Drugs* 2000; **60:** 1259–87.

MATERIAL FOR THE PRIMARY CARE PHYSICIAN

Bedell AW, Cady RK, Diamond ML et al. Patient-centered strategies for effective management of migraine. Primary Care Network, 2000.

Dowson A. Treating facial pain and nonmigraine headache. *Prescriber* 2001; **12:** 85–9.

Dowson AJ, Cady RK. *Rapid reference to migraine.* Mosby: London; 2002.

Dowson AJ, Gruffydd-Jones K, Hackett G et al. *Migraine: key facts. Essential information from MIPCA.* Richmond: Synergy Medical Education; 1998.

Dowson AJ, Gruffydd-Jones K, Hackett G et al. *Migraine management guidelines.* London: Synergy Medical Education; 2000.

Lipton RB, Stewart WF. *Using disability assessment to improve migraine care.* 3rd Edition, 1999. Available from www.migraine-disability.net.

Silberstein SD, Lipton RB, Goadsby PJ. *Headache in clinical practice.* Oxford: Isis Medical Media; 1998.

MATERIAL FOR THE PATIENT

Lipton RB, Stewart WF. *Managing your migraine. A guide for people with migraine.* 1999. available from www.migraine.org.uk and www.migraine-disability.net.

Wilkinson M, MacGregor A. *Understanding migraine & other headaches.* Banbury: Family Doctor Publications; 1999.

LIST OF PATIENT QUESTIONS

INDEX

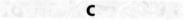

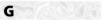

G

H